From   blic Health to Wellbeir

From Public Health to Wellbeing

The New Driver for Policy and Action

Edited by

Paul Walker

and

Marie John

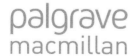
palgrave
macmillan

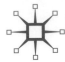
First published 2012 by
PALGRAVE MACMILLAN

Palgrave Macmillan in the UK is an imprint of Macmillan Publishers Limited,
registered in England, company number 785998, of Houndmills, Basingstoke,
Hampshire RG21 6XS.

Palgrave Macmillan in the US is a division of St Martin's Press LLC,
175 Fifth Avenue, New York, NY 10010.

Palgrave Macmillan is the global academic imprint of the above companies
and has companies and representatives throughout the world.

Palgrave® and Macmillan® are registered trademarks in the United States,
the United Kingdom, Europe and other countries

ISBN 978–0–230–27885–1

This book is printed on paper suitable for recycling and made from fully
managed and sustained forest sources. Logging, pulping and manufacturing
processes are expected to conform to the environmental regulations of the
country of origin.

A catalogue record for this book is available from the British Library.

A catalog record for this book is available from the Library of Congress.

10   9   8   7   6   5   4   3   2   1
21 20 19 18 17 16 15 14 13 12

Printed and bound in Great Britain by
CPI Antony Rowe, Chippenham and Eastbourne

Contents

List of Figures and Tables

Figures

Tables

Foreword

Wellbeing risks becoming one of the most overworked and ill-used words in the socio-political lexicon. Perhaps it was always so. The potent attraction of the desire to achieve it as the panacea sought to remedy the vagaries and challenges of the human condition lends itself to manipulation in political dogma; invokes it as an epitome of spiritual and religious yearnings; philosophizes it as the ultimate good for society and the fulfilment of the hedonic treadmill that carries us through life. A principal theme of this well-crafted book advocates placing the achievement of wellbeing by the individual and society, where it should be, as the principal objective of government and the community at large. What frustrates this laudable objective from being realized? The very nature of the wellbeing concept and its subjective elements defies attempts at its characterization, definition and measurement. There has been a lack of academic rigour for a robust analysis of its essential determinants in the individual person and in society. It needs to be unscrambled from 'happiness' which, though a cardinal component of wellbeing, is continually hijacked by the popular press, heralded as the solution to economic woes and degraded in a proliferation of revenue-seeking tawdry 'self-help' books.

The authors of this book confront these issues head on. The book is primarily aimed at first degree and masters students pursuing courses related to wellbeing, whom it will serve well. However, the information it imparts, the wide range of pertinent topics its chapters address in a coherent, cogent and constructive manner, and the welcome, well-substantiated case it advances for wellbeing as the driver for policy and action make it essential reading for a much wider constituency. Those involved in formulating and evaluating policy aimed at limiting social inequality and eliminating health inequalities will, in particular, benefit. The role and importance of the pursuit of wellbeing across the full span of the life course is eloquently articulated. Moreover, this book is not merely an academic treatise; the authors labour hard to offer solutions whereby wellbeing can be more effectively promoted, nurtured and sustained in a variety of settings. Intriguingly, the final chapter looks at a society in the not too distant future where securing the wellbeing of the population is the accepted norm and its pursuit the desirable goal of social policy – thus, wellbeing in all policies! It is a world in which we would all like to live.

Professor Sir Mansel Aylward, CB, FFPM, FFOM, FFPH, FRCP
Chair of Public Health Wales
Director of Centre for Psychosocial and Disability Research
School of Medicine, Cardiff University, UK

Acknowledgements

This book is the culmination of more than ten years of pondering on the meaning and import of wellbeing, and of discussions during this period with a wide range of colleagues in the former Dyfed Powys Health Authority, the National Public Health Service for Wales, PHA Cymru, the Welsh national branch of the UKPHA, the Socialist Health Association and at the University of Glamorgan. The number of individual colleagues who have influenced our thinking or contributed in some other way are legion, but those who have had a particularly important influence and/or made a significant contribution include Hannah John, Malcolm Ward, Gareth Davies, Gareth Williams, Amanda Reid, Antony Lewis, William Ritchie, Steve Clinton, Caroline Whittaker, and David and Hilda Smith.

The editors are grateful to the authors and publisher of *Policies and Strategies to Promote Social Equity in Health* by G. Dahlgren and M. Whitehead (Stockholm: Institute for Futures Studies, 1991) for permission to reproduce Figure 1.1; also thanks to Bristol City Council for Figure 2.3; Gallagher Estates for Figures 4.1, 4.3 and 4.4; the Town and Country Planning Association for Figure 4.2; Taylor & Francis for Figures 8.1 and 8.3, originally from Arnstein, S. (1969), 'A Ladder of Citizen Participation' in the *Journal of the American Institute of Planners*, vol. 35(4); the Institute of Public Health in Ireland for Figure 9.1; and the British Museum and Steve Haslam for the cartoon in Figure 10.1. Every effort has been made to contact all the copyright-holders, but if any have been inadvertently omitted the publishers will be pleased to make the necessary arrangement at the earliest opportunity.

Notes on the Contributors

Duncan Holtom is Head of Research at the People and Work Unit. Before joining the Unit, he worked as a Research Associate at the University of Queensland and the University of Wales, Swansea, where he also completed his PhD and Masters degrees.

Marie John has a nursing background and her passion for keeping people well was engendered following a post introducing a Health Promotion Group in a Trust. A Master of Science Degree in Health Promotion and Health Education consolidated this interest and led to a post with Health Promotion Wales. For the past twenty years held a post as a Senior Lecturer in Health Promotion and Public Health within a university setting. She retired in 2010.

Alan Joyner is a Fellow of the Royal Institution of Chartered Surveyors, a Fellow of the Royal Town Planning Institute, and holds Diplomas in Town Planning and Public Administration. Before joining the private sector, he was the Director of Planning, Transportation and Environmental Services at South Gloucestershire Council. He has presented numerous papers at conference events and seminars, written articles for professional journals, and appeared on local television and radio programmes to discuss town planning issues.

Sarah Lloyd-Jones is the Director of the People and Work Unit, an independent Welsh charity that uses action research techniques to explore socio-economic inequalities and their impacts, and ways of tackling inequalities. Her recent research includes a longitudinal study of the experiences of young adults who left school with no qualifications.

Marcus Longley was educated at the Universities of Oxford, Cardiff and Bristol, and held a variety of managerial and planning posts in the NHS in England and Wales during the 1980s and 1990s before joining the Welsh Institute for Health and Social Care, University of Glamorgan, at its inception in October 1995. He was appointed to a personal Chair at the University in 2006, and became Director of the Institute in 2008. He has held several advisory positions, including to the House of Commons Welsh Affairs Select Committee, the Welsh Local Government Association, and the Older People's Commissioner, and is a Board member of Consumer Focus Wales.

Gemma Pates is a psychologist and vocational rehabilitation specialist working in the NHS in Wales on the rehabilitation of people with acquired brain injury. She has research interests in the role of the psychological contract and wellbeing at work.

Richard Pates is a Consultant Clinical Psychologist and Independent Consultant. Formerly Clinical Director of NHS addiction services in Cardiff, member of ACMD and chair of the Welsh Advisory Committee on substance misuse. He is also the editor of the *Journal of Substance Use*, author of many papers, contributions to edited volumes and books.

Mike Ponton is a part-time Senior Fellow with the University of Glamorgan. His NHS posts included Chief Executive of Health Promotion Wales. As an official with the Welsh Assembly Government, he developed health policy and, latterly, was Director of the Welsh NHS Confederation. Mike retired in 2010.

Dafydd Thomas is the Coordinator of the Wellbeing Wales Network. He has worked in the voluntary and public sectors for over fifteen years on community, environmental and health issues. He is a member of the Physical Activity and Nutrition Network Wales, the All Wales Mental Health Network and is a Director of Timebank Wales.

Paul Walker is a medically qualified public health specialist with more than forty years' experience working for the National Health Service, local government and academe, latterly in Wales.

List of Abbreviations

ACMD	Advisory Council on the Misuse of Drugs
BPR	business process re-engineering
CHC	Community Health Councils
CSDH	Commission on Social Determinants of Health
CSLS	Canadian Centre for the Study of Living Standards
CUA	Cost-utility analysis
EWDs	Excess Winter Deaths
GNH	Gross National Happiness
GNP	Gross National Product
HDI	Human Development Index
HIA	Health Impact Assessment
HSE	Health and Safety Executive
HTA	health technology assessment
HUDU	Health Urban Development Unit
IEWB	Index of Economic Wellbeing
IQOLA	International Quality of Life Assessment
IRM	integrated resource management modelling
IT	information technology
MEW	measure of economic welfare
NHS	National Health Service
NICE	National Institute for Health and Clinical Excellence
OWB	objective wellbeing
PCT	Primary Care Trusts
PHC	Primary Health Care
PROMs	Patient Reported Outcome Measures
QALYs	quality adjusted life years
QLIs	quality of life indicators
RDA	Regional Development Agency
RIA	Regulatory Impact Assessment
RRC	Resilience Research Centre
RTPI	Royal Town Planning Institute
SCR	Scottish Centre for Regeneration
SMEs	small and medium sized enterprises
SWB	subjective wellbeing
UN	United Nations
UNCRC	United Nations Convention on the Rights of the Child
WHO	World Health Organization
WIHSC	Welsh Institute of Health and Social Care
WISP	Weighted Index of Social Progress

Introduction

Paul Walker

This book documents the evolution of public health thinking and practice, and of the conceptions of wellbeing, as well as the increasing realization of their convergence and congruence. For Cicero, the health of the people was the highest law. It is our contention that wellbeing is a more powerful, transparent and all-embracing framework than public health and that, today, it is the wellbeing of the people that should be the highest law.

It is no accident that all the authors work in Wales, which has strongly promoted the wellbeing notion through its landmark health, social care and wellbeing strategy initiative launched in 2003. Unsurprisingly, therefore, many of the examples given relate to Wales. However, this is not to imply that nothing relevant is happening elsewhere and appropriate reference is made to developments in the other countries of the United Kingdom and beyond.

The book's multi-authorship, with several different professional backgrounds represented, reflects the multifaceted nature of wellbeing. Some authors are academics; others are practitioners working in the public, voluntary and private sectors. We advocate a new wellbeing agenda based on ideas summarized from existing knowledge and evidence, and on some fresh thinking of our own.

The book is aimed principally at first degree and masters students pursuing courses in public health, health and wellbeing, health improvement/health promotion, social science and social work, town and country planning, public administration and policy studies. We envisage that it might also be of interest to members of the policy analysis and development communities, as well as to the general public.

Chapters 1 and 2 give the reader a foundation from which to explore the remaining chapters, introducing and analyzing the history and recent evolution of public health and wellbeing, with explanations of key terms, landmark developments and descriptions of current discourse.

The remaining chapters look at how wellbeing is impacting on current thinking and policy in a variety of contexts. Those chosen are not intended to be comprehensive or necessarily representative of all possible options. Rather, they have been selected because of their current policy salience. Two chapters look at major public sector institutions, the National Health Service and local government; two focus on specific age groups, children, and young persons and older people; two look at settings, the workplace and the community; and two more look at partnership working as the necessary platform for delivering wellbeing and at a particular policy area, substance misuse, which is perceived as beset with prejudice and muddled thinking and in need of radical reform adopting the wellbeing framework.

Chapter by chapter summary

Chapter 1 charts the development of public health thinking and action from ancient times to the present; identifies the 1946 World Health Organization (WHO) definition of health as a landmark broadening of the scope of conceptions of public health to include a subjective element and to encompass social factors; describes the developing wider determinants agenda initiated by the Black Report of 1980; and documents the main challenges facing public health in the new millennium.

Chapter 2 traces the origin and evolution of the development of the wellbeing concept from Aristotle and the Stoics to the present day; identifies some of the landmarks in the philosophical, theological, political, psychological and social policy discourse on the concept; charts its growing prominence and application over the last 20 years; explores its meaning in psychological terms; reviews approaches to measuring it and to applying it as the unifying framework and final common pathway for social policy. The chapter concludes by tracing the birth of wellbeing promotion out of the positive psychology movement.

Chapter 3 describes and analyzes why the wellbeing concept – whilst seemingly attractive to those concerned with health care policy because of the impact of unsustainable growth in demand and other pressures, plus a growing intellectual curiosity about better ways of defining the purpose of public policy generally – has failed to make much impact in the National Health Service (NHS). The chapter concludes by suggesting that the adoption of the wellbeing concept in the health care and other arenas will ultimately depend upon its perceived robustness and its measurability.

Chapter 4 examines what the promotion of a high degree of wellbeing could mean conceptually for spatial planning. It traces the history of town planning, and identifies lessons that can be drawn from the past to influence policies to be adopted and the services delivered by local authorities in the future. It explores how sustainable development is central to the UK planning system and how closely it relates to wellbeing; and it describes the role of partnership working between local government and other agencies in pursuing the sustainable wellbeing agenda.

Chapter 5 looks at why societies are particularly concerned about the wellbeing of children and young people and how protecting the wellbeing of children has come to be seen as important, both in its own right and as an investment in the future. It examines what constitutes wellbeing for children and young people, and considers why the wellbeing of children and young people has risen up the political agenda and in popular imagination. It looks at the dichotomy between society's wish to protect the wellbeing of the vulnerable child yet protect its own, and the extent to which the state can enable wellbeing and protect against illbeing.

Chapter 6 explores the concept of wellbeing in relation to older people and the challenges faced by society from their growing numbers. The particular factors that affect the wellbeing of older people are discussed with some insights into the effects of physical ageing. The chapter also examines the role and importance of partnership working between the many agencies involved in delivering wellbeing for older people.

Chapter 7 looks at wellbeing in the workplace, which has taken centre stage on the political agenda and has driven a fundamental rethink in UK public health and welfare policy. It explores some of the contextual influences that have shaped the modern workplace, influenced individual experience of work and necessitated policy reform.

Chapter 8 explores the links between community development and community wellbeing, and discusses what community development, community engagement and community wellbeing actually mean and also how it is possible to combine them. The chapter looks at different community engagement techniques that promote wellbeing, and concludes by considering what needs to happen at local and national government levels to make wellbeing interven tions happen as a matter of routine, rather than as exceptional instances of good practice.

Chapter 9 reviews the current state of understanding of collaboration in the form of partnerships, alliances and networks. From a theoretical perspective, informed by recent action research focused on improving multi-agency collaboration in Wales, it looks at the contexts and conditions under which collaborative activity can flourish; and explores how effective collaboration can be sustained.

Chapter 10 describes the use and abuse of mind altering substances, including alcohol through the ages and in different cultural contexts. It evaluates current global prohibitionist drug policy in terms of human rights legislation and in the context of the WHO Ottawa Charter. It concludes by stating the case, in terms of individual and community wellbeing, for the abandonment of current global prohibitionist policy in favour of some form of regulated legalization.

Chapter 11, which concludes, identifies lessons learned from the preceding chapters; provides a critique of the wellbeing concept advanced by key modern authors; and identifies the minimum actions deemed necessary to advance the wellbeing agenda. This chapter does some crystal ball gazing on what the NHS and local government might look like in 25 years' time, assuming an enthusiastic and wide ranging adoption and application of the wellbeing framework and all that flows from it.

Bibliography

Cicero (1914) *De Finibus Bonorum et Malorum* (On Ends), H. Rackham, trans. Loeb, Classical Library. Cambridge: Harvard University Press.

Welsh Assembly Government (2003) *Health, Social Care and Well-being Strategies*. Cardiff: Welsh Assembly Government.

On Public Health and Wellbeing

Paul Walker

This chapter summarizes the development of public health systems and thinking from ancient times to today. It identifies some of the critical events that have significantly influenced this development, some current issues and some of the challenges that could shape its evolution. It concludes by exploring the congruence of the concepts of health and wellbeing.

Introduction

The word 'health' is derived from the Old English *hæl* meaning wholeness, of being whole, sound or well with overtones of holy, sacred and healing.

Public health has been defined in many ways (p. 12) but its two distinctive characteristics are that it deals with the prevention of disease/illness, rather than cure or healing; and that its focus is populations rather than individuals. The population in question can be as small as a handful of people or as large as all the inhabitants of several continents – as for instance, in the case of pandemics.

The evolution of public health thinking and practice

Before 1840: of plagues and empiricism

Public health is a modern concept, although it has roots in antiquity. From the beginnings of human civilization, it was recognized that polluted water and lack of proper waste disposal spread vector-borne diseases.

Around ten thousand years ago, when people began to move from being nomadic hunter-gatherers to living a more settled farming lifestyle, the risks to health changed. Increased contact with people and animals and their waste products generated new problems. But, while the nature of both disease and good health was little understood, some ancient civilizations evolved rituals in which cleanliness and a healthy lifestyle were central. Usually religious in origin, some of these behaviours were also effective public health measures. In ancient Babylon, for example, religious teaching forbade drinking wells being dug near cemeteries and rubbish dumps. Cleanliness was also associated with religion in ancient Egypt, where an emphasis on washing had obvious public health benefits. The Chinese developed the practice of variolation (inoculation) following a smallpox epidemic around 1000 BC.

The ancient Greeks understood some of the links between lifestyle, the environment and health. Advice on diet, exercise and cleanliness is found in the works of Hippocrates (*On Airs, Waters and Places*). Inevitably, these Greek ideas influenced the Romans. While the ancient Greeks instituted some central control of public health, as had the rulers in ancient China and India, this greatly increased under the Romans, who believed that cleanliness would lead to good health and that prevention of illness was as important as its cure. From empirical observations, they made links between causes of disease and methods of prevention, as a consequence of which they developed a sophisticated system of public health infrastructure throughout the Roman Empire. Such observations led them to believe that ill health could be associated with, amongst other things, bad air, bad water, swamps, sewage, debris and lack of personal cleanliness. Their response was to provide clean water through aqueducts, to remove the bulk of sewage through the building of sewers and to develop a system of public toilets throughout their towns and cities. Personal hygiene was encouraged through the building of public baths.

The decline of the Roman Empire was accompanied by the loss of much of the public health infrastructure. However, in the Near East parts of the rising Islamic Empire developed health care services and public health schemes. Baghdad opened its first hospital in 800 AD and, by the year 1000 AD, had sixty of them. A number of cities also had public baths and sewage systems. In some ways, it is difficult to conceive of a more public health-friendly religion than Islam, which strongly advocates healthy behaviour. The *Quran* and the *hadith* (teachings and sayings of the Prophet Muhammad) offer numerous directives about maintaining health at community, family and individual levels.

From the eleventh century, growing international trade stimulated urbanization in western Europe, with a resulting rise in the prevalence of communicable diseases. Leprosy was especially widespread and laws enforcing the isolation of sufferers were passed throughout the medieval period. Such powers were expanded in the wake of the Black Death and the subsequent waves of plague that recurred over several centuries. The development of the practice of quarantine in this period also helped to mitigate the effects of other infectious diseases.

With the decline in the toll of the plague in the eighteenth century there was less need for strict public health measures. At the same time, an interest in the underlying health of populations developed. Counting and valuing – characteristics of trading nations with growing empires – were now applied to populations. Censuses, disease statistics, birth rates and bills of mortality marked the earliest beginnings of epidemiology: the science of public health (Porter, 1999).

By the late 1700s, Britain was evolving into the first industrialized nation – a revolution that created public health challenges of a type still faced today as industrialization spreads around the world. Although this new age brought medical advances, it occurred within a social climate of *laissez faire*, where little thought was given to ensuring that people were healthy, clean or well-housed. However, the cholera pandemic that devastated Europe between 1829 and 1851 stimulated government action leading to measures such as regulating the location of cemeteries which were based on the then current miasmatic theory of disease. Other public health interventions included latrinization; the building of sewers; the regular collection of garbage, followed by incineration or disposal in a landfill site; the provision of clean water and the draining of standing water to prevent mosquitoes breeding.

1840 to 1980: from microbes to lifestyle

Reports by social reformers such as Edwin Chadwick revealed the extent of the public health crisis in Britain. He drafted the revisions of the Poor Laws and was subsequently the administrator for the Poor Law Commissioners. It was the failure of the workhouse system, however, that led Chadwick to public health. His *Report on the Sanitary Condition of the Labouring Population of Great Britain*, published in 1842, argued that the primary cause of pauperism and misery was not poverty or rampant capitalism, but filth. To him, the water queue, the dung heap and the cesspool were the causes of moral decline, fever and death. His arguments were a counterpoint to the more radical visions of William Cobbett (Cole, 1924); the Chartists; and Friederich Engels (Henderson, 1976), as expressed in *The Condition of the Working Class in England*, published in 1844, and in the *Communist Manifesto* of 1848. Work, wages and food were rejected as remedies for pauperism in favour of water and sewerage systems. The notion that poverty itself was the cause of illness was, for Chadwick, unthinkable (Hamlin, 1998).

Public pressure for health reform, combined with Chadwick's advocacy on sanitation, prompted the government to pass its first Public Health Act in 1848 which, over the following decades, stimulated the growth of public health bureaucracies armed with increasingly strong powers. A German physician, Johann Peter Frank , had at this time developed the concept of Medical Police (*Medizinische Polizei*), comprising a state administered system of health inspectors with powers to quarantine, disinfect and cleanse with the aim of promoting population growth, a healthy labour force and fit military recruits (Lesky, 1976). This policing model was a major influence during the nineteenth century in Britain as elsewhere, to which the development of the key role of the Medical Officer of Health bears witness.

The impact of these developments in sanitation was, however, extremely limited: by the start of the twentieth century, slum housing was still a prominent feature of many cities, and the poor physical condition of Boer War recruits bore witness to the deprivations endured by large sections of the population.

In 1700, there were only seven towns outside London with a population greater than 10,000 (Clark and Slack, 1976) but, with the influx of workers and their families into the rapidly industrialized towns during the 1800s, this number increased significantly, leading to overwhelming problems of overpopulation. Ashton and Seymour (1988) describe the findings of Dr Duncan, Liverpool's first Medical Officer of Health, who wrote of one third of the population of Liverpool living in the cellars of back-to-back houses with earth floors, no ventilation or sanitation, and as many as 16 people in one room. The infrastructure of these communities had not been built to withstand such a population explosion and, in the early nineteenth century, 'the problems of environmental degradation, disease and human misery reached massive proportions and were in evidence across large tracts of Britain' (Webster, 1990).

To provide professional leadership for sanitary reform, local authorities appointed Medical Officers of Health, medical practitioners with appropriate training in the then new science of public health. Over time, local authorities gained new roles and, by the 1930s, the Medical Officer of Health's empire had grown to include environmental health, district nursing, community midwifery, health visiting, school health, maternal and child health, mental health, welfare and the former Poor Law hospitals. At the height of local authorities' power and independence, Medical Officers of Health were important people with considerable influence within organizations.

The modern study of the social determinants of health can be said to have begun with the writings of Rudolph Virchow (Koch, 1882) and Friedrich Engels (Henderson, 1976), and the creation of social medicine during the mid-nineteenth century. Virchow and Engels not only made the explicit link between living conditions and health, but also explored the political and economic structures that create inequalities in the living conditions that lead to health inequalities.

The scientific underpinning of public health – epidemiology – was established by John Snow's identification of a polluted public water well as the source of a cholera outbreak in Golden Square, London in 1854 (Snow, 1855).

As the prevalence of infectious diseases in the developed world decreased during the twentieth century, public health began to place greater focus on chronic diseases such as cancer and heart disease.

A key development of the 1920s was the publication of the Dawson Report: 'Interim Report on the Future Provision of Medical and Allied Services of the Consultative Council on Medical and Allied Services' (MOH, 1920). Lord Dawson was 'convinced that preventive and curative medicine cannot be separated on any sound principle, and in any scheme of medical services must be brought together in close coordination' (MOH, 1920: 6). He proposed that health care in a given district should be based upon 'Primary Health Centres', which he termed 'institutions equipped for services of curative and preventive medicine to be conducted by the general practitioners of that district' (MOH, 1920: 6). These centres were to be supported by secondary health centres and teaching hospitals, which would deal with difficult cases requiring special treatments and/or expert diagnosis. This pattern of provision provided the framework on which the National Health Service (NHS) was constructed in 1948.

A particularly prescient focus of the Dawson Report was on the value of physical culture as a vital necessity to the health of the nation (MOH, 1920: 30).

Not long after the publication of the Dawson Report, but probably not influenced by it, the Peckham Experiment was initiated (Barlow, 1988). This was a study into the nature of health. It lasted from 1926 to 1950 and was conducted by Drs George Scott Williamson and Innes Hope Pierce, both of whom refused to divide souls from bodies or to divide bodies into sets of distinct medical specialities.

Healthy Living Centres are a recent derivative of the long-defunct Peckham Experiment. These are based on the recognition that determinants of poor health in deprived areas include economic, social and environmental factors that are outside the influence of conventional health services. Several more recent projects have also been based on a holistic approach to health and a commitment to partnership with patients. For example, the Bromley by Bow Centre links health, education, arts and the environment. Activities include a community education programme, a food cooperative, complementary therapies and exercise classes. In Bristol, Knowle West Health Park is planned to include a new health centre, family centre, dance studio, community café, jogging track and community gardens.

The dramatic increase in average life span during the twentieth century is widely attributed to public health achievements, such as vaccination programmes and the control of infectious diseases, effective safety policies (such as motor vehicle and occupational safety), improved family planning, the chlorination of drinking water, smoke-free measures and programmes designed to decrease chronic disease. In the aftermath of the Second World War, the further expansion of government involvement in health culminated with the emergence of the welfare state. In Britain, this was characterized by the introduction of financial and medical assistance from the cradle to the grave, the most significant component of which was the launch of a National Health Service in 1948.

At the same time, the World Health Organization (WHO), created in 1946, developed its landmark definition of health as 'a state of complete physical, mental, and social wellbeing and not merely the absence of disease or infirmity'. This definition, which remains unchanged, has been much criticized for its lack of practical application. It also lacks internal coherence in envisaging wellbeing in both subjective terms (mental wellbeing) and objective terms (physical and social wellbeing). Conceptually, however, it marked the first explicit equating of health with wellbeing in modern times.

Public health initiatives have now moved beyond national boundaries with the WHO launch of extensive international campaigns – often combining health education with practical activities such as vaccination. Under its auspices, the global eradication of smallpox was achieved in the 1980s and the global eradication of poliomyelitis is currently well-advanced.

The Lalonde Report (1974), *A New Perspective on the Health of Canadians*, is considered to be the first modern government document in the Western world to acknowledge that our emphasis upon a biomedical health care system is wrong, and that we need to look beyond the traditional health care (sick care) system, if we wish to improve the health of the public. It proposed a new health field concept with four major determinants of health: human biology, environment, lifestyle and health care organization. The report emphasized individuals' roles in changing their behaviours to improve their health, and was groundbreaking in identifying health inequalities as a major issue.

In the UK, 1974 was a watershed in public health that saw the transfer of many public health functions and their associated personnel from local government to the NHS (Draper *et al.*, 1976). This resulted in a loss of confidence within the public health community that was apparent from the lack of progress in developing the public health agenda over the next twenty years. This was only partially countered by the implementation of the recommendations of the Acheson Report of 1988.

The establishment of the Faculty of Community Medicine as a faculty within the Royal Colleges of Physicians of the UK in 1972 reinforced the medical domination of the public health function which impeded the involvement of other disciplines so important to developing the so called wider determinants agenda by at least two decades.

Two notable publications of the 1970s were Ivan Illich's *Medical Nemesis* (1975) and Thomas McKeown's *The Role of Medicine: Dream, Mirage or Nemesis* (1976), both of which promoted the view that improvements in health in the nineteenth and twentieth centuries had little to do with medical interventions, and more to do with social conditions and the actions of individuals and society.

The Declaration of Alma-Ata, adopted at the WHO International Conference on Primary Health Care in Kazakhstan in 1978, expressed the need for urgent action by all governments, all health and development workers, and the world community to protect and promote the health of all the people of the world. It was the first international declaration underlining the importance of primary health care. The primary health care approach has, since then, been accepted by member countries of the WHO as the key to achieving the goal of 'Health for All'. The first section of the declaration reaffirms the WHO definition of health, and seeks to include the social and economic sectors within the scope of attaining health through *intersectoral collaboration*; it also reaffirms health as a human right.

The Healthy Cities project was established by the WHO in 1985 as a test bed for Health for All and, in the UK, achieved some success in promoting intersectoral collaboration between local authorities, health authorities, voluntary agencies and even the private sector. Liverpool was the site of one particularly active Healthy City project, and the county of Norfolk uniquely applied the same concept in a large rural county in the 1990s with some success (Norwich Health Authority, 1990). The programme continues today with about 8000 cities worldwide now engaged, Cardiff being amongst the most recent signatories.

Since 1980: from inequalities in health to social determinants

Inequalities in health

Inequalities in health have been noted since the time of Hippocrates: Chadwick, in his *Report on the Sanitary Condition of the Labouring Population of Great Britain* (1842), documented the wide discrepancy in longevity between occupational groups in different parts of England. However, seeing such groups as more than just an interesting finding of descriptive epidemiology is a recent phenomenon: I received my public health training in 1970/71 in Edinburgh without any reference whatsoever to this issue.

Sir John Brotherston, in his 1975 Galton Lecture, identified various occupations as a cause for concern, which was echoed the following year in the Labour government's landmark document 'Prevention and Health: Everybody's Business' (DHSS, 1976). In this lecture, Sir John Brotherston identified inequalities in health as a cause for concern.

In August 1980, the UK Department of Health and Social Security published the Report of the Working Group on Inequalities in Health, also known as the Black Report. It demonstrated in great detail the extent to which ill health and death were unequally distributed among the population of Britain, and suggested that these inequalities had been widening rather than diminishing since the establishment of the NHS in 1948. The Report concluded that these inequalities were not mainly attributable to failings in the NHS but, rather, to social inequalities influencing health (such as income, education, housing, diet, employment and conditions of work). In consequence, the Report recommended a wide strategy of social policy measures to combat inequalities in health. The findings and conclusions of this landmark report were amplified and developed by Margaret Whitehead in *The Health Divide* (1987).

The ensuing decade saw a growing rhetoric but a commitment to real action is a latter day phenomenon. The turning point was 1998, with the publication of the Independent Inquiry into Inequalities in Health Report (Acheson, 1998). As with earlier reports, including the Black Report, this inquiry demonstrated the existence of health disparities and their relationship to social class. Among the Report's findings were that, despite an overall downward trend in mortality between 1970 and 1990, the upper social classes experienced a more rapid mortality decline. The report contains 39 policy suggestions, in areas ranging from taxation to agriculture, for ameliorating health disparities.

In 2002, the Chancellor of the Exchequer commissioned Sir Derek Wanless, a former banker, to undertake a review on prevention and the wider determinants of health in England, and on the cost-effectiveness of action that can be taken to improve the health of the whole population and to reduce inequalities. He envisaged three possible future scenarios, the slow uptake, solid progress and the fully-engaged (where members of the public were fully engaged with measures to improve the public health). He suggested that, for this to happen, people needed to be supported more actively to make better decisions about their own health. This included providing a single accessible source of advice on health issues.

In 2005, the WHO established the Commission on Social Determinants of Health (CSDH) under the chairmanship of Sir Michael Marmot. The Commission reported in 2008. It was recommended that national governments should develop and implement strategies and policies suited to their particular national context aimed at improving health equity. In the UK, the English and Scottish governments have undertaken so-called Marmot Reviews in response to this recommendation that propose evidence-based strategies for reducing health inequalities from 2010.

Since the 1980s, the focus of public health has shifted from individual behaviours and risk factors to population-level issues such as inequality, poverty, and education. Modern public health is concerned with addressing health determinants across a population, rather than simply advocating individual behaviour change, recognizing that health is affected by many factors including the environment, genetics, income, educational status and social relationships, the so-called 'wider' or 'social' determinants of health. Among those who were instrumental in effecting this shift in focus were those in the health promotion profession, the evolution of which, out of the narrower paradigm of health education, was a feature of the 1980s.

The WHO Regional Office for Europe defined health promotion as the process of enabling people to increase control over and improve their health. In addition to methods to change lifestyles, the WHO also advocated legislation, fiscal measures, organizational change, community development and spontaneous local activities against health hazards.

Two years later, the WHO launched the Ottawa Charter for Health Promotion at the first international conference for health promotion. This identified five action areas for health promotion:

- building healthy public policy;
- creating supportive environments;
- strengthening community action;
- developing personal skills; and
- re-orientating health care services toward prevention of illness and promotion of health.

The WHO also proposed three basic strategies for health promotion:

- advocacy;
- enablement; and
- mediation.

A Committee of Inquiry into the future development of the public health function (Cmd 289) was established and reported in 1988. This was undertaken in the light of continuing concerns among public health practitioners about their role following the NHS reorganization of 1974, and in the wake of a spectacular failure of public health personnel to respond appropriately to a traditional public health challenge: a salmonella outbreak in a large psychiatric hospital in the north of England. Public health was thus defined, in a much wider context than before, as the science and art of preventing disease, prolonging life and promoting health through the organized efforts of society. This definition reveals key ideas embedded in much contemporary public health, identifying partnership and multidisciplinary working, collaboration, an evidence-based approach and the breadth of action from population health gain through to the provision of health care services. It also illustrates the complex and contested nature of public health.

Dahlgren and Whitehead (1991) described a social ecological theory of health. In this, they attempt to map the relationship between the individual, their environment and disease (Figure 1.1). Individuals are at the centre, with a set of fixed genes. Surrounding them are influences on health that can be modified:

- the first layer is personal behaviour and ways of living that can promote or damage health – individuals are affected by friendship patterns and the norms of their community;
- the next layer is social and community influences, which provide mutual support for members of the community in unfavourable conditions; they can, however, also provide no support or have a negative effect;
- the third layer includes structural factors – housing, working conditions, access to services and provision of essential facilities.

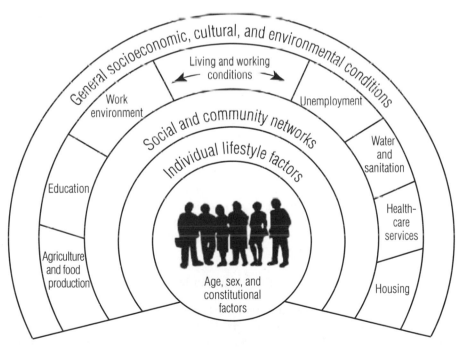

Figure 1.1   The relationship between the individual, the environment and disease

Source: Dahlgren and Whitehead (1991), reproduced with the kind permission of the Institute for Futures Studies, Stockholm

In his seminal text *The Strategy of Preventive Medicine* (1992), Geoffrey Rose summarized the challenges to public health, as he saw them:

> and that means a new partnership between the health services and those whose decisions influence the determinants of incidence. The primary determinants of disease are mainly economic and social, and therefore its remedies must also be economic and social. Medicine and politics cannot and should not be kept apart.

The 'new public health'

The term 'new public health' (Holman, 1992) has been current since the 1980s but, confusingly, has been used to denote different versions of recent public health. Lifestyle public health of the 1970s, in the wake of the Lalonde Report, emphasized individual responsibility for the prevention of ill health. Limitations of this approach led to a new formulation in the 1980s that focused on environmental concerns and health inequality. The so-called 'new public health' movement in the UK was, in part, aimed at recreating the link between environmental health and public health doctors, which had been broken by the NHS reorganization in 1974. Ashton and Seymour's book *The New Public Health* (1988) became the movement's landmark publication. The impact on health of the environment and of a range of social factors was seen as crucial by organizations such as the Public Health Alliance, which was established in 1987. More recently, there has been an increasing emphasis on the role of secondary prevention by clinicians and of genetics.

The evolution of public health and public health thinking can be seen in three phases:

- the phase of empirical observation characteristic of Ancient Greece and Rome;
- the phase of empirical action based on such observations which was initiated by Rome and characterized the subsequent period until the middle of the 19th century; and
- the scientific phase which can be subdivided into the microbial phase focused on communicable diseases, sanitary measures and vaccination and immunization, and the multi-factorial/wider determinants phase initiated by the WHO with its Health for All movement and given a fillip by the publication in the UK of the Black Report (DHSS, 1980) and *The Health Divide* (Whitehead, 1987).

An alternative view categorizes this evolution in four stages (Figure 1.2):

- *Stage 1*, lasting until the mid-twentieth century, focused on the environment, interpreted broadly to include flora and fauna;
- *Stage 2*, from 1950 to 1980, where health care was remarkably short, where health care was seen as important;
- *Stage 3*, from 1980 to 1990, where lifestyle was the dominant theme; and
- *Stage 4*, the current position, where the socioeconomic environment comprising the wider/social determinants, is seen as pre-eminent.

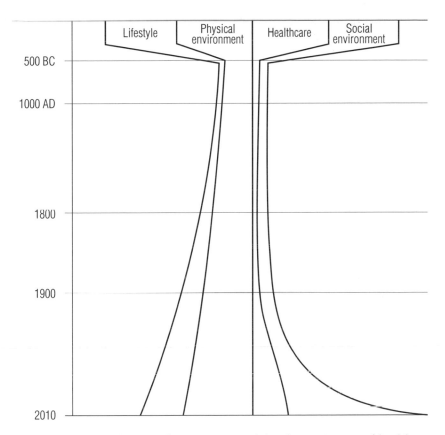

Figure 1.2   The evolution of conceptions of the determinants of health

Stage 4 represents a gradual shift to the adoption of the concept of wellbeing, with its all-embracing canvas of determinants, and the acceptance of the congruence of the concepts of health and wellbeing conceived by the WHO in 1946, with its landmark definition.

Current issues

Medical hegemony

Interest in public health, quite understandably, first developed among members of the medical profession. So it was that early public health practitioners, including the first Medical Officers of Health in the UK, were also practising clinicians in the latter case – general practitioners usually.

Well into the nineteenth century, this state of affairs persisted throughout the developed world. In the UK, in spite of the major contribution to public health by lawyer Edwin Chadwick, the state of medical hegemony continued until very recently. Only on the eve of the new millennium was the speciality of public health at last opened up to non-medical practitioners.

In fact, medical hegemony was strengthened in the 1970s when public health, then termed very deliberately 'community medicine', was accepted as a medical speciality with the establishment of the Faculty of Community Medicine under the umbrella of the Royal Colleges of Physicians of the United Kingdom. In reaction to this, the non-medical discipline of health promotion evolved out of health education and expanded during this period.

Despite current rhetoric about the decline of medical hegemony, there is a continuing demarcation between medical and non-medical public health appointments. Posts such as regional directors of public health and consultants in communicable disease control remain restricted to medically qualified candidates. Non-medical directors of public health at Primary Care Trust (PCT) level earn significantly less than their medical colleagues doing the same job.

The contested nature of public health

As already suggested, public health is a contested concept. It is presented and used in a variety of ways by public health practitioners, researchers and commentators. In the UK at least, it has even changed its name from time to time. In the first half of the 1900s, the term 'state medicine' was coined as an alternative, emphasizing the collectivist nature of much public health action. In the 1970s, the term 'community medicine' was adopted, following a lead from Morris (1969) focusing on the group nature of the recipients of such action.

Some of the most influential or interesting definitions or accounts of public health include:

Public health is the science and the art of preventing disease, prolonging life and promoting physical health and efficiency through organised community efforts for the sanitation of the environment, the control of community infections, the education of the individual in principles of personal hygiene, the organisation of medical and nursing service for the early diagnosis and preventative treatment of disease, and the development of social machinery which will ensure to every individual in the community a standard of living adequate for the maintenance of health (Winslow, 1920).

What we, as a society, do collectively to assure the condition in which people can be healthy (Institute of Medicine, 1988).

The science and art of preventing disease, prolonging life and promoting health through organised efforts of society (Acheson, 1988).

'Government intervention as public health' involves public officials taking appropriate measures pursuant to specific legal authority ... to protect the health of the public ... The key element of public health is the role of government – its power and obligation to invoke mandatory or coercive measures to eliminate a threat to the public's health (Rothstein, 2002).

Society's obligation to assure the conditions for people's Health (Gostin, 2001).

Childress *et al.* (2002) prefer to list features or aspects of public health:

Public health is primarily concerned with the health of the entire population, rather than the health of individuals. Its features include an emphasis on the promotion of health and the prevention of disease and disability; the collection and use of epidemiological data, population surveillance, and other forms of empirical quantitative assessment; a recognition of the multi-dimensional nature of the determinants of health; and a focus on the complex interactions of many factors biological, behavioural, social and environmental in developing effective interventions.

The diversity of these definitions is noteworthy – some being very broad in their nature and scope, whilst others focus on a more narrow range of considerations. Some are highly normative; others more or less descriptive. Some even contain detailed guidance as to how the relevant ends of public health are to be achieved. The Winslow definition, though written in 1920, has probably been the most influential.

Separation from local government

One of the major impediments to developing the public health agenda in the UK has been the separation of the main parts of the public health function from local government since the reorganization of the NHS in 1974. Active collaboration between the NHS and local authorities on an agreed public health programme is the obvious remedy. However, in the main this has not happened. Differences in culture and issues of organizational language have resulted in a virtual stand-off between local authorities and health service organizations, even though the list of local government functions and services that act to improve the health and wellbeing of the local population exceeds that of any other single public body.

In England, one development that has sought to improve collaboration is the joint appointment of Directors of Public Health by coterminous local authorities and Primary Care Trusts. It is generally felt that this has been helpful – necessary, even – but certainly not sufficient to bring about the level of collaboration required.

Involving the general public

Another area where public health has failed is in involving the public in decision-making. It would appear that there is a tendency among public health professionals to want to shape public behaviour, rather than be informed by it. Put another way, they favour the expert/evidence model of public health practice, rather than the leader/development model.

Working with Community Health Councils (CHCs) to inform the public on health issues and to seek their views was seen as a key part of the job of community physicians in the immediate aftermath of the 1974 NHS reorganization. It is fair to say, however, that not all CHCs were very interested in public health, as distinct from hospital and general practice health care; and not all public health practitioners understood the fundamental importance of CHCs. The net result was that, overall, public involvement in public health decision-making and activity was negligible. When CHCs were replaced in England, the situation did not improve. Community Health Councils have been retained in Wales, but there is no clear evidence that this has had the effect of improving the public's involvement in the public health agenda.

And what was true of the statutory public health sector was, unhappily, equally true of the voluntary sector public health bodies such as the UK Public Health Association, the Royal Society for the Promotion of Health and the Royal Institute of Public Health and Hygiene, which saw their main role as representing public health practitioners of various kinds, rather than representing or advocating for the general public.

Health care primacy

One issue that arguably dominates all other factors is that of the overriding tension between health care and health, and the continuing imbalance between them. The NHS continues to dominate the health policy agenda, as it has done without interruption since its founding. The result is that health care has been consistently prioritized over public health. As Coote (2007: 138) has it: 'Health policy has been so thoroughly skewed towards illness and services that a visitor from outer space could be forgiven for assuming that the main role of government in this field is to fund and manage vast armies of doctors and nurses in hospitals up and down the country, all striving to repair sick bodies'.

One development that many in the public health community pressed for was the establishment of a Minister for Public Health to give some political weight to the development of public health policy, and to protect it from the customary depredations of the health care/sickness agenda. The last Labour government did, in fact, respond to this by creating such a post, but did not take the necessary steps of giving the post cabinet status. More importantly, the post of Minister for Public Health was not relocated away from the Department of Health to some more appropriate Department, such as the Cabinet Office or the then Office of the Deputy Prime Minister.

In its NHS White Paper 'Equity and Excellence: Liberating the NHS' (Department of Health, 2010) proposals and its stated intentions in respect of the public health function, the coalition government seems to want to dilute this health care domination of the policy agenda.

Links with primary care

Although the Dawson Report (1920) promoted the idea of close working between general practitioners and public health practitioners, and the Peckham Pioneer Health Centre experiment was essentially about promoting community health and wellbeing from a health centre setting, collaboration between primary care and public health has been, in the main, a non-event. The National Health Act 1946 did not include prevention in the general practitioner contract and, even when anticipatory care was included many years later, this tended to be individually oriented clinical anticipatory care, rather than community focused. During the 1960s, when a major health centre building programme was launched, the result was decreased rather than increased collaboration, because general practitioners were suspicious that Medical Officers of Health would seek to coordinate all community-based services. Many influential general practitioners, including Pickles (1929) and Julian Tudor Hart (1988), have argued for primary care to exploit its public health potential and for the public health content of primary care to be explicitly recognized. Mant and Anderson (1985) even suggested that community medicine (as public health was known at that time) and general practice should move towards integration.

With the increasing recognition of the importance of the social determinants of health, the potential role for general practitioners and other primary care staff to look beyond the individual patient consultation to what is happening in the community where their registered patients live, and to apply community development and other techniques to make the community more health-promoting more salutogenic, should be being exploited, developed and researched (Walker, 2009). Sadly, this is not the case and the changes proposed by the coalition government NHS White Paper would appear to make this even less likely in the future.

Cuba has adopted a system where primary care physicians and nurse teams have responsibility not only for delivering health care to their patients, but also for the health of geographically defined populations (Evans, 2008).

Future challenges

In 2002, the European Public Health Association looked at the future of public health and identified the following main challenges (Noack, 2006):

- the future of public health can only be achieved if the whole of society invests in it; building partnerships is essential to this;
- the long-term benefits of public health should be taken seriously by policy-makers;
- public health should form an integral part of the political agenda in all sectors;
- public health policy should be based on assets, rather than disease;
- research remains a solid basis for the development of public health practice and policy;
- research should focus on the needs of policy and practice;
- researchers should learn how to interact with politicians and practitioners;
- innovative ways to promote health should be encouraged;
- the future of public health should be based on the principle 'think globally, act locally', with policies set up at national or international level and

implementation at local level adapted as appropriate to local needs and circumstances.

Looking more parochially, the major public health challenges facing the UK relate to smoking – still an issue, though declining in importance; obesity; alcohol misuse; sexually transmitted infections/teenage pregnancies; and, dwarfing all these, inequalities in health. Drug misuse is also an issue, though more in relation to the evidence-blind, prejudiced approach to policy adopted by the government – the antithesis of a public health approach – than in relation to the scale of the problems caused by drug use, which pale into insignificance in comparison to those caused by alcohol misuse, for example. These challenges are also faced to a greater or lesser degree by other developed countries.

Adopting a global perspective, in *The Public Health System in England* Hunter *et al.* (2010) add climate change to this list. They conclude that what is needed is a new public health movement, a revival of the spirit of Alma-Ata, to meet these challenges, and suggest that the WHO European Region Health Charter adopted in 2008 in Tallinn could signal such a revival.

To me, it is clear that the immediate challenge to the public health community is to ditch the muddled thinking and internal conflicts, and the preoccupation with occupational positioning of the past, and embrace the new wellbeing paradigm. The public health community has the skills and experience to provide leadership in this new world, but only if it does not look back.

From public health to wellbeing: the path for progress

To the ancient Greeks, health (*hygeia*) and wellbeing (*eudaimonia*) were distinct. In Aristotle's discourse on the meaning of *eudaimonia*, health was a necessary but not sufficient component of *eudaimonia*. To the more practically-minded Romans, wellbeing and health were the same: *salus*.

Until 1946, generally speaking, health was defined in objective terms as the absence of disease within a Cartesian framework where mind and body were conceived as entirely separate. In that year, however, the fledgling WHO defined health as much more than this: a complete state of physical, mental and social wellbeing. The source of this ground-breaking definition is not clear, and no definition was offered of the term 'wellbeing'. It could be argued that it is conceptually confusing to conflate mental wellbeing (a subjective state of mind) with physical and social wellbeing (clearly, objective states). However, the 1946 WHO definition established that, in essence, health and wellbeing were one and the same thing.

With the dawning and development of the wider determinants perspective on health in the wake of the Alma-Ata Declaration in 1978 and the Black Report in 1980, there began a gradual moving away from the medical model of health as the absence of disease to an all-embracing concept that increasingly matched the 1946 WHO formulation, with an increasing focus on social wellbeing and the social determinants of health. This effectively took health out of the hands of doctors and the health care community, and handed it to the whole of society.

In spite of this broadening of perspective, the link between health and well-being was not acknowledged by the public health community, and the use of the term 'wellbeing' in public health discourse was rare. It did gain currency, but in other disciplinary communities – particularly in the field of sustainable development and Agenda 21. (Agenda 21, the outcome of the United Nations Conference on Environment and Development held in 1992, is a comprehensive blueprint of action to be taken globally, nationally and locally by organizations of the United Nations, governments and major groups in every area in which humans directly affect the environment.)

The reticence of the public health community in adopting Agenda 21 is a puzzle; adopting it would allow it to spread its sphere of interest and involvement to, quite literally, every aspect of public sector, voluntary sector and even private sector activity. Naturally, the converse is also true, and it could be that putting up the 'keep out' notice in respect of its own bailiwick is, ultimately, more important to the public health community than expanding its empire by responding positively to the challenge and opportunity of the wellbeing concept. The territorial imperative is very strong, particularly in those who feel insecure!

However, if 'health' and 'wellbeing' mean the same thing, does it matter which term is used; does using the composite term 'health and wellbeing' help? To most people, including politicians and policy-makers, the term 'health' is still strongly linked to doctors, nurses and health care, and is thus severely restricted in its field of vision. Without adding the term 'wellbeing', the term 'health' tends to have the traditional 'disease focus'. It could be argued that' in time' this myopia will be overcome as an understanding of the significance of the wider/social determinants grows. However, the current issues and future challenges to public health are with us now and need to be tackled – now.

Adopting the word 'wellbeing' instead of 'health', it is suggested:

- would make it much easier to engage local authorities, non-health-related disciplines and the public;
- would make partnership working easier, at least for local authorities and the voluntary sector;
- could weaken the impediments of medical and health care hegemony;
- might even, paradoxically, make it easier for general practitioners to take on a local community development role; and
- would make engagement with the sustainable development and inequalities agendas much easier at local, national and global levels.

Adopting Wanless' (2002) terminology, it is posited that the use of the word 'wellbeing' would be more likely to secure *the fully engaged scenario* in tackling current issues and future challenges than using the word 'health'. Without a fully engaged scenario, progress will be slow and piecemeal, at best.

It is tempting to conclude that the two terms should co-exist, with each being used in the appropriate context – 'wellbeing' when dealing with the social/wider determinants agenda, and 'health' in conversation with the health care community and those involved in the traditional public health fields of public protection and health care improvement. This would be misguided, however, because there is a growing realization that, within the NHS and public health, there is a state of what might be described as 'institutional disease-ism'; that is, a focus on disease entities, rather than the subjective experience of them. This is not to say that a focus on diseases is no longer important, only that modern enlightened health care and public health practice requires a balanced consideration of both objective and subjective elements. If using the composite term 'health and wellbeing' makes it easier for this to happen, this is reason enough to use it. And, lest it be thought that a focus on wellbeing as well as health might compromise the extent to which measurement is possible, as demonstrated in Chapter 2, subjective and objective wellbeing are measureable – often using the same metrics as are used to measure objective and subjective health.

Bibliography

Acheson, D. (1998) *Independent Inquiry into Inequalities in Health*. London: HMSO.

Acheson, D. (1988) *Public Health in England: The Report of the Committee of Inquiry into the Future Development of the Public Health Function*. London: HMSO.

Ashton, J. (1999) 'Past and Present Public Health in Liverpool', in S. Griffiths and D.J. Hunter (eds), *Perspectives in Public Health*. Abingdon: Radcliffe Medical Press

Ashton, J. and Seymour, H. (1988) *The New Public Health*. Milton Keynes: Open University Press.

Barlow, K. (1988) *Recognising Health*. McCarrison Society: 74–82.

Bendiner, E. (1995) 'Sara Josephine Baker: Crusader for Women and Children's Health', *Hospital Practice* (United States), 30(9): 687.

Brotherston, J. (1975) 'Inequality: Is it Inevitable?', in C.O. Carter and J. Peel (eds) (1980) *Equalities and Inequalities in Health*. London. DHSS.

Chadwick, E. (1842) *Report on the Sanitary Condition of the Labouring Population of Great Britain*, M.W. Flinn (ed.). Edinburgh: Edinburgh University Press.

Childress, J.F., Faden, R.R., Gaare, R.D., Gostin, L.O., Kahn, J., Bonnie, R.J., Kass, N.E., Mastroianni, A.C., Moreno, J.D. and Nieburg, P. (2002) 'Public Health Ethics: Mapping the Terrain', *Journal of Law, Medicine and Ethics*, 30(2): 170–8.

Cicero (1914) *De Finibus Bonorum et Malorum* [On the Ends of Good and Evil], H. Rackham (trans.), Loeb Classical Library (Cambridge: Harvard University Press). Latin text with old-fashioned and not always philosophically precise English translation.

Clark, P. and Slack, P. (1976) *English Towns in Transition 1500–1700*. London: Oxford University Press.

Cole, G.D.H. (2011 [1924]) *The Life of William Cobbett*. Abingdon: Routledge.

Cooper, Laurence (1999) *Rousseau, Nature and the Problem of the Good Life*. Pennsylvania: Pennsylvania State University Press.

Coote, A. (2007) 'Labour's Health Policy: The Cart before the Horse?', *Soundings*, 35(1): 37–47.

Dahlgren, G. and Whitehead, M. (1991) *Policies and Strategies to Promote Social Equity in Health*. Stockholm, Institute for Futures Studies.

DHSS (1980) *The Report of the Working Group on Inequalities in Health*, Chaired by Sir Douglas Black. London: DHSS.

DHSS (1976) *Prevention and Health: Everybody's Business*. London. HMSO.

Draper, P., Grenholm, G. and Best, G. (1976) 'The Organisation of Health Care: A Critical Review of the 1974 Reorganisation of the NHS', in D. Tuckett (ed.), *An Introduction to Medical Sociology* (2003). London: Tavistock Publications.

Evans, R.G. (2008) 'Thomas McKeown, meet Fidel Castro: Physicians, Population Health and the Cuban Paradox', *Healthcare Policy*, 3(4): 21–32.

Gostin, L. (2002) *Public Health Law and Ethics: A Reader*. Berkeley: University of California Press.

Hamlin, C. (1998) *Public Health and Social Justice in the Age of Chadwick: Britain, 1800–1854*. Cambridge: Cambridge University Press.

Dyfed Powys Health Authority (2002) 'Health and Well-Being in Dyfed Powys: The Annual Report of the Director of Public Health for Dyfed Powys Health Authority'. Dyfed Powys Health Authority.

Norwich Health Authority (1990) 'Healthy Norfolk People, Norwich and District: On the State of its Health', *Department of Public Health Medicine*, October.

Henderson, W.O. (1976) *The Life of Friedrich Engels*. London: Cass.

Hippocrates (1938) *On Airs, Waters, and Places*. Translated and republished in *Medical Classics*, 3: 19–42.

Holman, C.D'A.J. (1992) 'Something Old, Something New: Perspectives on Five New Public Health Movements', *Health Promotion Journal of Australia*, 2(3): 4–11.

Hunter, D., L. Marks and K. Smith (2010) *The Public Health System in England*. University of Bristol: Policy Press.

Illich, I. (1974) *Medical Nemesis*. London: Calder & Boyars.

Institute of Medicine (1988) *The Future of Public Health*. Washington, DC: National Academic Press.

Koch, R. (1882) 'Die Atiologie der Tuberkulose' ['The Aetiology of Tuberculosis']. Berlin. *Klinischen Wochenschift*, 19: 221. Trans. and repr. in M. Pinner (trans.) (1913) *The Aetiology of Tuberculosis*. New York: National Tuberculosis Association.

Lalonde M. (1974) *A New Perspective on the Health of Canadians. A Working Document*. Ottawa: Government of Canada.

Lesky, E. (ed.) (1976) *A System of Complete Medical Police: Selections from Johann Peter Frank*. Baltimore, Maryland and London: Johns Hopkins University Press.

Mant, D. and Anderson, P. (1985) 'Community General Practitioner', *The Lancet*, 326(8464): 1114–7.

Masters, R. (ed.) (1978) *On the Social Contract, with the Geneva Manuscript and Political Economy by Jean-Jacques Rousseau*, Judith R. Masters (trans.). New York: St Martin's Press.

McKeown, T. (1976) *The Role of Medicine: Dream, Mirage or Nemesis*. London: Nuffield Provincial Hospitals Trust.

MOH (1920) Consultative Council on Medical and Allied Services, 'Interim Report on the Future Provision of Medical and Allied Services'. London: HMSO.

Morris, J.N. (1969) 'Tomorrow's Community Physician', *The Lancet*, 294(7625)(2): 811–16.

Noack, R.H. (2006) 'The Future of Public Health in Europe: Towards a More Active Partnership with WHO/EURO', *European Journal of Public Health*, 16(2), April: 226–8.

Pickles, W. (1951) 'Trends of General Practice: A Hundred Years in a Yorkshire Dale', *The Practitioner*, 167(1000): 322–9.

Porter, D. (1999) *Health, Civilization and the State: A History of Public Health from Ancient to Modern Times*. London: Routledge.

Rose, G. (1992) *The Strategy of Preventive Medicine*. Oxford: Oxford University Press.

Rosen, G.A. (1993) *History of Public Health*, expanded edn. Baltimore: Johns Hopkins University Press.

Rothstein, M. (2002) 'Rethinking the Meaning of Public Health', *Journal of Law, Medicine and Ethics*, 30: 144–9.

Snow, J. (1855) *On the Mode of Communication of Cholera*, 2nd edn. London: Churchill. Reproduced in *Snow on Cholera* (1936) New York, Commonwealth Fund; repr. (1965) New York: Hafner.

Swift, J. [1726, amended 1735] *Gulliver's Travels*.

Tudor Hart, J. (1988) *A New Kind of Doctor*. London: Merlin Press.

Walker, P. (2009) 'Tackling Inequalities through Primary Care', *National Association of Primary Care Review*, spring: 25–7.

Wanless, D. (2002) *Securing Our Future Health: Taking a Long-Term View*. London: Department of Health.

Webster, C. (ed.) (2001) *Caring for Health: History and Diversity*, 3rd edn. Buckingham: Open University Press.

Webster, C. (1990) *The Victorian Public Health Legacy: A Challenge to the Future*. Birmingham: Public Health Alliance.

White, K.L. (1991) *Healing the Schism: Epidemiology, Medicine, and the Public's Health*. New York: Springer-Verlag.

Whitehead, M. (1987) *The Health Divide: Inequalities in Health in the 1980s*. London: Health Education Council.

Winslow, E.A. (1920) 'The Untilled Fields of Public Health', *Science*, 51(1306): 23–33.

World Health Organization (2008a) *The Tallinn Charter: Health Systems for Health and Wealth*, WHO European Ministerial Conference on Health Systems: Health Systems, Health and Wealth, Tallinn, Estonia, 25–27 June. Copenhagen: WHO.

World Health Organization (2008b) *Closing the Gap in a Generation. Final Report of the Commission on Social Determinants of Health*. Geneva: WHO.

World Health Organization (1985a) *Health for All in Europe by the Year 2000: Regional Targets*. Copenhagen: WHO.

World Health Organization (1985b) *The Ottawa Charter for Health Promotion. Health Promotion*, 1(4): iii–v. PLACE: WHO.

World Health Organization (1978) *Report on the International Conference on Primary Care*, Alma-Ata. Geneva: WHO.

World Health Organization (1946) *Constitution*. Geneva: WHO.

Wellbeing: Meaning, Definition, Measurement and Application

2

Paul Walker

This chapter traces the origin and evolution of the wellbeing concept from Aristotle and the Stoics to the present day. It identifies some of the landmarks in the philosophical, theological, political, psychological and social policy discourses on the concept, and reviews attempts to measure it and to apply it as a driver of social policy. It concludes by tracing the birth of wellbeing promotion out of the Positive Psychology movement.

Origins and development of the concept of wellbeing

A major landmark in the development of the wellbeing concept enshrined in the questions 'What is the nature of a good life?' and 'What is it that makes life desirable?' occurred in Ancient Greece when it was much debated by philosophers – notably, Aristotle – as *eudaemonia* (Inwood and Gerson, 1998).

Eudaimonia is a central concept in ancient Greek ethics. Some philosophers believed *eudaimonia* to be the highest human good – the best, noblest, and most pleasant thing in the world, according to Aristotle – and were concerned with studying ways of achieving it. In his *Nicomachean Ethics*, Aristotle states that *eudaimonia* means doing and living well (Broadie, 1991): the really difficult question is to specify just what sort of activities enable one to live well. Aristotle presents various popular conceptions of the best life for human beings. The candidates that he mentions are a life of pleasure, a life of practical activity and a philosophical life.

The standard English translation of *eudaimonia* is 'happiness'. However, it is important to note that happiness does not entirely capture the meaning of the Greek word. One important difference is that happiness often connotes being, or tending to be, in a certain pleasant state of consciousness. In contrast, *eudaimonia* is a more encompassing notion than happiness, since events that do not contribute to one's experience of happiness may yet affect one's *eudaimonia*.

Because of this discrepancy between the meaning of *eudaimonia* and happiness, some alternative translations have been proposed. W.D. Ross (Stout, 1967) suggests 'well-being' and John Cooper (1997) proposes 'flourishing'.

The word *wele*, cognate with today's words 'wealth' and 'wellbeing', surfaced in the English language in about 1250 and meant 'happiness' and also 'prosperity'. In its original meaning, very significantly, the intention matters more than the present state or circumstances.

Wellbeing in modern theological, philosophical, political, psychological and social policy discourse

It is noteworthy that discourse on wellbeing and related concepts more or less disappeared, at least in Europe, during the period of Catholic Christian hegemony, apart from in the writings of theologians such as Thomas Aquinas and Augustine of Hippo. It resurfaced during the Enlightenment, the great contribution of which to discourse lay in the validation of pleasure. It accorded legitimacy to pleasure not as occasional binges, mystical transports or blue-blooded privilege, but as the routine entitlement of people at large to pursue the senses, not just purify the soul; and to seek fulfilment in this world and not only in the next (Porter, 2000: 260).

The promotion of wellbeing was included, in concept, in the 1776 US Declaration of Independence (Bailyn, 1992), although the word 'happiness' was used rather than 'wellbeing'. Among Enlightenment figures who addressed the issue of happiness from various perspectives were Thomas Paine in his *Rights of Man* (Keane, 1995), Jean Jacques Rousseau (Cooper, 1999) and the architects of the French Revolution (Doyle, 1981). Utilitarian philosophers in eighteenth- and nineteenth-century England identified pain and pleasure as the only intrinsic values in the world, and Jeremy Bentham's Felicific Calculus (Bentham, 1789) put happiness on the philosophical agenda in the mid-nineteenth century. To Marx (Avineri, 1968), species being (or happiness) was the pinnacle of human nature. This is understood to be a type of self-realization or self-actualization brought about by meaningful work. But, in addition to engaging in meaningful work, self-actualized individuals must also own the products of their labours and have the option of doing what they will with those products.

Attention to the concept of *eudaimonia* and ancient ethical theory more generally enjoyed a revival in the twentieth century. Nietzsche (1909), in the 'Metamorphoses' section of *Thus Spoke Zarathustra*, sets out a three-part meditation and the process of spiritual transformation through stages represented by the camel, the lion and the child, that characterizes his vision of a flourishing life. A life-affirming, child-like spirit is crucial to happiness, health, and wellbeing, with the individual discovering the joy of life and the innocence of creation.

The concept of wellbeing and its achievement is implicit in most Utopian literature, and in developments such as Ebenezer Howard's Garden City movement (1898).

Looking at the impact of the wellbeing concept on social policy discourse in the UK and globally, there were two landmark events during the 1940s: the publication of the Beveridge Report, and the definition of health promoted by the World Health Organization (WHO).

The Report of the Inter-Departmental Committee on Social Insurance and Allied Services chaired by William Beveridge and published in 1944 identified five Giant Evils in society: squalor, ignorance, want, idleness and disease. The Report went on to propose widespread reform to the system of social welfare to address these. These five issues comprise what we now recognize as the key domains of objective wellbeing (p. 32).

An event with more global impact was the definition of health as a complete state of physical, psychological and social wellbeing by the fledgling WHO in 1946. This, in effect, equated health with wellbeing. (The relationship between health and public health with wellbeing is discussed in Chapter 1.)

An interest in wellbeing was a feature of the twentieth-century liberalism and the socialism of figures such as Anthony Crosland (1956) who, in *The Future of Socialism*, asks if happiness should be the primary objective of social democratic politics.

In recent decades, researchers in a range of fields have initiated a major effort to improve understanding of happiness and other psychological aspects of wellbeing. After fitful beginnings in the 1960s, this work started to take off with the pioneering research of Ed Diener (1984) and others in the 1980s. The literature has grown explosively since the beginning of the new millennium – particularly since Martin Seligman (2003) and Mihaly Csikszentmihalyi (1990), among others, inaugurated the Positive Psychology movement. In 2005, Nettle reported that over 3000 studies on the topic had been published since the 1960s.

Besides positive psychology, there are now the often overlapping fields of subjective wellbeing research, happiness studies, hedonic psychology, *eudaimonic* psychology, behavioural economics and neuro-economics, among others. And, most recently, a growing body of work has driven a more sophisticated understanding of wellbeing – drawing on economics, psychology and political philosophy.

Sen, in *Commodities and Capabilities* (1999), adopts an approach to human wellbeing that emphasizes the importance of freedom of choice, individual heterogeneity and the multidimensional nature of welfare.

A recent key event in the penetration of the wellbeing concept into establishment thinking in the UK was the Local Government Act 2000. Part 1 of this Act provides local authorities with a discretionary power (the Well Being [sic] power) to undertake any action to promote or improve the social, economic and environmental wellbeing of their area, though no definition is given of 'wellbeing'. The main aim of the Act was to overcome some of the barriers to innovative action by local authorities imposed by the *ultra vires* rule; and to encourage crosscutting action within local authorities themselves, and between local authorities and other local agencies such as the NHS.

In the wake of the enactment of this wellbeing power in Wales, the Welsh Assembly Government published 'Well Being in Wales' in 2002 and, in the following year, initiated its landmark Health, Social Care and Wellbeing Strategy agenda. 'Well Being in Wales' builds on the foundation set by 'Better Health, Better Wales' (Welsh Office, 1998), a green paper that set out the Welsh Assembly Government's aims for sustainable health through collaborative action, and which identified a wide range of social and environmental factors impacting on the health and wellbeing of the people of Wales.

Significantly, 'Well Being in Wales' went further than 'Better Health, Better Wales' in identifying wellbeing as a core aim. It identified a high level of wellbeing as a feature of strong and vibrant communities, and an individual's or community's wellbeing as depending on several factors including:

- people's interests and the extent to which there is a sense of engagement in, and access to, the community;
- happiness and feelings of confidence and self-esteem;
- health and safety;
- security – financial and otherwise;
- the services, facilities and opportunities available to everyone, and people's comfort and overall quality of life.

This was followed in 2003 by the Welsh Assembly Government's launch of its Health, Social Care and Wellbeing Strategy agenda, of which the key features are partnership working, and an integrated and multidisciplinary approach to local authority and NHS strategic planning. It placed a legal responsibility on local authorities and local health boards for joint needs assessment, strategy formulation and implementation; and imposed on them a duty of collaboration with other public sector, voluntary sector and private sector organizations in fulfilling this responsibility.

Wellbeing: what is our current understanding of the meaning of the word and the concept?

'Wellbeing' is a state of mind or consciousness that, for Aristotle and the Ancient Greek philosophers, comprised both affective and cognitive components, each being necessary but not sufficient by itself. Whether wellbeing or *eudaimonia* includes an element of the third component of the psyche – conation – is a moot point. 'Conation' is the personal, intentional, deliberate, goal-oriented or striving component of motivation, the pro-active (as opposed to reactive or habitual) aspect of behaviour. It is an absolutely critical element, if an individual is to engage successfully in self-direction and self-regulation: it is virtually ignored in the literature.

So, wellbeing as a state of mind – that is, subjective wellbeing (SWB) – can be construed as comprising three components: affect, cognition and, putatively, conation. The affective or hedonic component, commonly termed 'happiness', refers to both the presence of positive affect and the absence of negative affect. It is guided by emotions and feelings. The cognitive component is an information-based appraisal of one's life, for which people judge the extent to which their life so far measures up to their expectations and resembles their envisioned ideal life. It approximates to Maslow's (1980) notion of self-actualization.

The relative importance of these three components almost certainly varies from individual to individual, from society to society, and with different time horizons affect being more important for short-term wellbeing and cognition more important for long-horizon wellbeing.

Relationship to other similar measures

There are currently several other concepts closely related to wellbeing widely cited in the social policy literature. These include:

- *quality of life*, which tends to relate to constituents of the physical environment rather than a state of mind;
- *life satisfaction*, which relates mostly to the cognitive aspect of wellbeing and is, as the term suggests, a summation over a long period of time;
- *happiness*, as we have seen, relates mainly to the affective element of wellbeing;
- *mental health/positive mental health* similarly relates mainly to the affective element;
- *welfare*, as with quality of life, tends to relate to the external environment; and
- *wellness*, another widely used term that tends to be used by the alternative medicine community and relates to the affective element of wellbeing.

The relationships between some of these different concepts are explored by Nettle (2005) who distinguishes three levels of happiness:

- W1: the first level comprises momentary feelings of joy and pleasure;
- W2: the second level comprises judgements about feelings wellbeing and satisfaction;
- W3: the third level comprises quality of life, and relates to flourishing and fulfilling one's potential.

Level 1 is the most immediate, sensual and emotional, more reliably measured and more absolute; whereas level 3 is more cognitive, more relative, more moral and political, and involves more cultural norms and values. Level 2 represents the middle ground.

Figure 2.1 is a diagrammatic representation of the three time frames of wellbeing. This figure also indicates a notional distribution of mental states between affect and cognition for each timeframe, with cognition predominating at the W3 and W2 levels, and affect at the W1 level.

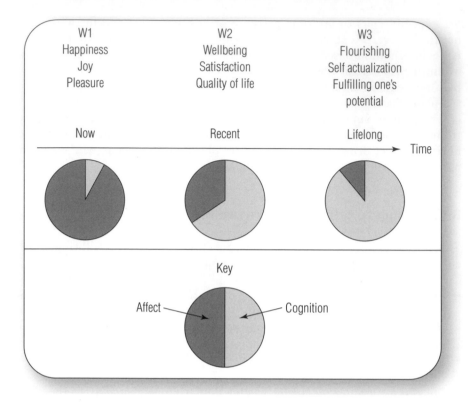

Figure 2.1   The spectrum of wellbeing

Another interesting and related concept is that of 'flow', a rhythm of absorption and satisfaction that Mihaly Csikszentmihaly (1990) equates with happiness.

Modern definitions

Today, the term 'wellbeing' is used increasingly frequently by a wide range of organizations, scholars and political bodies in a range of contexts, but there is no single consistent definition, as can be seen from the following:
UNICEF (2007: 1) suggests that:

> wellbeing means having the basic things you need to live and being healthy, safe and happy.

The OECD (2006: 9) contends that:

> individuals derive wellbeing from the satisfaction of their wants according to their own preferences.

Others have noted:

> Important non-economic predictors of the average levels of wellbeing of societies include social capital, democratic governance, and human rights. Finally, wellbeing is related to health and longevity (Diener and Seligman, 2004).

> The emphasis upon the effort to live a life well together with others and on wellbeing outcomes that are continuously generated through conscious and subconscious participation in social, economic, political and cultural processes (McGregor *et al.*, 2008).

> Wellbeing stems from the degree of fit between individuals' perceptions of their objective situations and their needs, aspirations or values (Andrews and Whithey 1976; Campbell *et al.*, 1976).

The key themes that are reflected in all these definitions are health, security (both economic and physical), and the ability to engage on social, political and cultural levels.

Robert Prescott-Allen (2001) distinguishes the concept of human wellbeing from ecosystem wellbeing, which he defines as a condition in which the ecosystem maintains its diversity and quality – and, thus, its capacity to support people and the rest of life, and its potential to adapt to change and provide a wide range of choices and opportunities for the future. In his book, *The Wellbeing of Nations*, he endeavours to combine measures of both types of wellbeing in assessing global wellbeing and that of its individual nations. To him, sustainable development is simply a combination of human wellbeing and ecosystem wellbeing. Another way of looking at it is to conceive of sustainable wellbeing as wellbeing with a clear future dimension, concerned not only with wellbeing today and yesterday, but also with the wellbeing of future generations.

In 2006, the UK Government Whitehall Wellbeing Working Group developed a statement of common understanding of wellbeing for policymakers:

> Wellbeing is a positive physical, social and mental state; it is not just the absence of pain, discomfort and incapacity. It arises not only from the action of individuals, but from a host of collective goods and relationships with other people. It requires that basic needs are met, that individuals have a sense of purpose, and that they feel able to achieve important personal goals and participate in society. It is enhanced by conditions that include supportive personal relationships, involvement in empowered communities, good health, financial security, rewarding employment, and a healthy and attractive environment.

> Government's role is to enable people to have fair access now and in the future to the social, economic and environmental resources needed to achieve wellbeing. An understanding of the combined effect of policies on the way people experience their lives is important for designing and prioritising them.

Wellbeing as the underlying objective of all social policy

Geoffrey Rose (1992) introduced the concepts of proximal and underlying causes to public health discourse, with the aim of re-focusing the attention of policy-makers and politicians onto the reasons for behaviours that compromise health, rather than the behaviours themselves. Thus, smoking can be seen as an individual addictive behaviour where the immediate reason for taking up the habit is the strong psycho-active effect of nicotine. But smoking can also be seen as an individual's response to stress in their particular milieu. So, a more effective way to combat smoking is to improve people's conditions of living, rather than offer services that help them combat nicotine addiction, such as smoking cessation services.

A similar two-tier approach can be applied to the aims of social policy. Thus, there are the immediate or proximal aims of a particular policy and the underlying aims. To take housing policy as an example, the proximal aim of most housing policies is to improve the condition and/or security of tenure of an individual's living conditions. But the underlying aim is to improve the individual's wellbeing. This two-tier model can be applied to all aspects of social policy. From this, it becomes clear that the underlying aim, explicit or implied, of all social policy is to improve the wellbeing of the individuals/populations concerned. Thus, it follows that wellbeing can be conceived as the unifying concept for all social policy.

(An analysis of the factors affecting the penetration of the wellbeing concept within the NHS is included in Chapter 3.)

The epidemiology of wellbeing

Whatever definitions of wellbeing are used, there is a consensus that it is influenced by a myriad of factors. In all accounts, these include personal dispositions and social supports, life experiences and income. Genetics also plays a part, and how genetic inheritance interacts with the environment and shapes how well people cope with difficult life circumstances.

A report for the UK Prime Minister's Strategy Unit (2002) identified five factors that shape an individual's wellbeing:

- *genetics*: 40–50 per cent is genetically determined;
- *personality*: high intelligence, extroversion, optimism, high self-esteem, planning and organizational skills and low neuroticism;
- *physical attributes*: physical attractiveness for women and height for men;
- *gender*: women have marginally higher levels of satisfaction; and
- *age*: young people and older people experience higher levels of life satisfaction than the middle-aged (the U-shaped pattern).

Richard Easterlin (1974) developed what became known as the Easterlin Paradox, which argues that once wealth reaches subsistence level, its effectiveness as a generator of wellbeing is greatly diminished. Richard Layard

(2009) suggests, however, that, over the past fifty years, rising living standards have had some positive effects on overall happiness, but this has been offset by the negative effects of worsening human relationships, more broken families, more pressure at work and less cohesive communities. Johns and Ormerod (2007) show that recorded levels of happiness fluctuate from year to year but that there is no trend, either up or down, even though gross national product per head had shown a very clear upward trend at their time of writing.

Wellbeing tends to be lower in countries with higher inequality in income and wealth. The link between child wellbeing and income inequality is significantly stronger than the relationship between child wellbeing and absolute incomes (Wilkinson and Pickett, 2007).

A 2008 Eurobarometer survey of what people considered to be important across the 27 EU countries showed that health ranked highest (73 per cent of respondents) followed by love (44 per cent), work (37 per cent), peace (35 per cent) and money (32 per cent). The overwhelming importance attached to health is noteworthy.

Table 2.1 presents the factors that influence happiness derived from a poll conducted for the BBC in 2005.

Other documented associations include:

- *Race*: in the USA, African Americans have usually been found to experience lower subjective wellbeing than white people (Diener, 2009).
- *Education*: in the USA, there is evidence that the level of education has a small influence on subjective wellbeing, which appears to be more pronounced in women (Diener, 2009).
- *Life events*: unsurprisingly, good events are related to positive affect and bad ones to negative affect. There is evidence, however, that the ability to take control of life events affects their impact on subjective wellbeing, with even pleasant events lessening subjective wellbeing if they lead to a feeling of lack of control (Diener, 2009).

Table 2.1   Factors that influence happiness

Factor	Influence (%)
Health	24
Money and financial situation	7
Religious/spiritual life	6
Community and friends	5
Work fulfilment	2
A nice place to live	8
Partner/spouse/family relationships	47
Don't know/other	1

Source: Poll undertaken for the BBC by GfK NOP during October 2005. Results available at http://news.bbc.co.uk/nol/shared/bsp/hi/pdfs/29_03_06_happiness_gfkpoll.pdf.

Table 2.2   Happiness in the UK (2008/9)

Population group	Score (average on scale 1–7)
Age 15–24	5.28
Age 25–34	5.22
Age 35–44	5.10
Age 45–54	5.00
Age 55–64	5.34
Age 65 and over	5.49
No children at home	5.27
Children	5.17
Married	5.37
Single	5.16
Separated	4.74
Divorced	4.86
Not religious	5.15
Religious	5.31
Church of England	5.31
Roman Catholic	5.16
Full-time student	5.46
Worker	5.28
Unemployed	4.64
Lowest decile monthly incomes	5.05
Highest decile monthly incomes	5.45

Source: British Household Panel Survey 2008/9.

Table 2.2 gives the average happiness scores for a selection of population categories as measured in the British Household Panel Survey of 2008/9. The high score for those aged 65 years and over is remarkable, as is the low score for those who are separated.

Other determinants of wellbeing are discussed in various chapters in this book:

- Chapter 4 looks particularly at environmental factors;
- Chapter 5 looks at what affects the wellbeing of children and young people;
- Chapter 6 explores what impacts on the wellbeing of older people;
- Chapter 7 looks at what aspects of the workplace affect wellbeing; and
- Chapter 10 discusses the role of drugs and other psychoactive substances on individual and community wellbeing.

Can we measure wellbeing?

The western worldview is dominated by notions of progress. Progress is seen to be about making life better; that is, improving quality of life and wellbeing. Indicators are crucial to such progress because we cannot know, as a society, whether wellbeing or quality of life is improving unless we can monitor and measure any changes that take place. Policies, for example, are judged on how they affect relevant indicators.

As economies grow, societies tend to devote attention to measures that are most easily quantifiable and that have the clearest upward trajectory. In the wake of the recession, and against the backdrop of global imperatives to manage carbon dioxide emissions, there is a burgeoning interest in developing and testing new measures of success. The OECD's work through its global project on Measuring Social Progress is one focus of interest.

The breakthrough in devising ways to measure wellbeing came in the 1950s, when psychologists – who, until then, had been mainly interested in negative emotional states such as depression and anxiety – became interested in positive emotions and feelings of wellbeing. A great deal of effort has been devoted by the discipline of psychology to trying to measure the mental state that is wellbeing by means of a variety of instruments. This has resulted in what is known as the psychometric approach to measuring subjective wellbeing (SWB). A very simple approach would be to ask people directly whether they are happy and self-fulfilled, and that they indicate this by choosing a smiley/frowny face that represents how they feel. Technically, this is known as a single-item measure of SWB, of which there are many documented (Figure 2.2 offers an example). One of the shortcomings of single-item measures is their inability to assess separately the various dimensions of wellbeing. But, if a survey must be brief and cheap where only an overall indication of SWB is needed, a single global measure such as the smiley/frowny face array is defensible.

Local authorities currently carry out annual quality of life surveys of their populations and, in many cases, ask respondents to indicate on a five-point scale their satisfaction with services provided by them and with aspects of their life circumstances, including their levels of happiness and life satisfaction. Figure 2.3 is an extract from the survey questionnaire used by Bristol City Council in 2010.

Another approach is to ask people about their satisfaction with issues that research studies have identified as being felt to be important to people's sense of wellbeing, such as partner/spouse and family relationships, health and

Figure 2.2   An example of a single-item measure of subjective wellbeing

---

44. Taking all things together, would you say you are?
(Please tick 1 box)

Very happy   ☐
Quite happy   ☐
Not very happy   ☐
Not at all happy   ☐

45. All things considered, how satisfied are you with your life as a whole these days? (please circle a number)
1 means you are completely dissatisfied, 10 means you are completely satisfied

Dissatisfied   1   2   3   4   5   6   7   8   9   10   Satisfied

---

Figure 2.3   Part of the Bristol City Council quality of life survey question-naire (2010), reproduced with the permission of Bristol City Council

financial circumstances, economic wellness, environmental wellness, physical wellness, mental wellness, workplace wellness, social wellness and political wellness. An example of this approach is the SF-36, where questions are asked about such things as mental health, emotional state, social functioning and feelings of vitality. This approach delivers what are known as multiple-item measures of SWB.

Validation of both single-item and multiple-item scales which are self-reported can be done with reference to external non-self-reported criteria such as interviewer ratings, peer ratings, facial coding and other non-verbal measures.

Figure 2.4 is a diagrammatic representation of the factors, internal and external, impacting on the three time frames of SWB. It demonstrates that the external factors affecting SWB vary in their relative importance with time. The socio-economic environment is considered to be the most important factor for short-term wellbeing, with the power/control factor assuming much more importance with medium- and long-term wellbeing.

An alternative epidemiological approach is to identify determinants, corre-lates or associations of the state of mind of wellbeing and attempt to measure these, and so arrive at an indirect measure of wellbeing: objective wellbeing (OWB). Unlike SWB which can have three time horizons (W1, W2 and W3), OWB, by the nature of its construction, relates to the medium-term time hori-zon, W2. Figure 2.5 is a diagrammatic representation of some of the factors – those that are included in various UK indices of multiple deprivation – contributing to OWB.

Inevitably, there are approaches that contain elements of both SWB and OWB; for example, the Economist Intelligence Unit's quality-of-life index.

Figure 2.6, developed by the author for the magazine *Healthmatters* in 2009, endeavours to represent SWB in the form of the smiley/frowny face, and OWB in the form of the segments of the circle at a particular point in time,

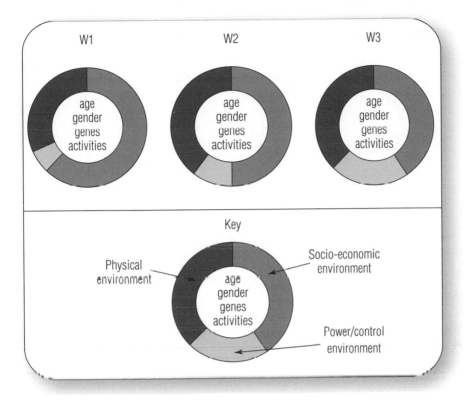

Figure 2.4   Factors impacting on subjective wellbeing

September 2009. Its aim was to chart the impact of the government's financial cutbacks on the national state of wellbeing. Figure 2.6 indicates that SWB was considered to be low (a medium frowny face) and, of the domains of OWB, those that were having the greatest impact were income and employment, both of which were in decline at that point.

There is a strong argument for using both kinds of measure in order to avoid the problem of adaptation where, for example, individuals report high wellbeing scores in the presence of disadvantage of various sorts, such as poverty leading possibly to inaction to tackle the poverty. Such action, seemingly sanctioned by looking only at the SWB scores, would do nothing to reduce inequalities in wealth, which is known to undermine population wellbeing.

Most of the many multifactor indices that have been developed to measure wellbeing comprise mainly measures of OWB.

In 2007, the report 'Local Wellbeing: Can We Measure It?' explored how wellbeing can be effectively measured at a local level by making maximum use of the current data framework set for local government by central government and the Audit Commission. The aim was to support local authorities in understanding local need, effectively measuring outcomes, tracking progress and informing decisions on resource allocation.

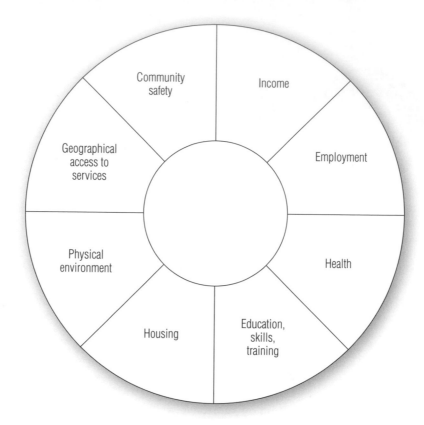

Figure 2.5   Factors impacting on objective wellbeing

It took as its starting point the international experience of other municipalities. The Young Foundation Report, *The State of Happiness* (2010), proposes a three-tiered approach for measuring wellbeing:

- *universal level*: a single item measure giving an overall and crosscutting picture of peoples lives;
- *domain level*: this measures outcomes with different thematic objectives – for example, health, education, community safety; and
- *targeted level*: this focuses on the underlying or protective factors that impact on people's wellbeing – for example, indicators associated with resilience, self-esteem and competency.

The Commission on the Measurement of Economic Performance and Social Progress (2008) – established by French President Nicolas Sarkozy and chaired by Nobel Prize-winning economist Professor Joseph E. Stiglitz of Columbia University – has identified three conceptual approaches to measuring quality of life. The first approach, closely linked to the utilitarian tradition, is based on the notion of SWB. The second approach, with strong links to philosophical concepts of social justice, is rooted in the notion of capabilities and focuses on

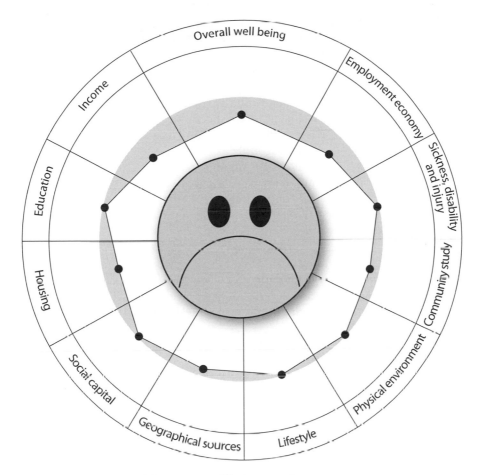

Figure 2.6   The *Healthmatters* wellbeing graph

the individual's ability to pursue and realize the goals that they value. The third approach, developed within the economics tradition, is based on the notion of fair allocations. The basic idea is to weight the various non-monetary dimensions of quality of life in a way that respects people's preferences.

Three crosscutting issues are identified by the Commission as deserving special attention. The first is to detail the conditions relating to inequalities in the various dimensions of life, rather than just the average for each country. There are many inequalities, and each is significant in itself.

The second is to better assess the relationship between the various dimensions of quality of life. Some of the most important policy questions relate to how developments in one area (e.g. education) affect developments in others (e.g. health status, political voice and social connections), and how developments in all fields are related to those in income.

The third crosscutting issue is to aggregate the rich array of measures in as parsimonious a way as possible. The issue of aggregation is both specific to each feature of quality of life (as in the case of measures that combine mortality and morbidity in the health field) and more general, requiring the valuation and aggregation of the achievements in various domains of life, both for each person and for society as a whole.

Rather than focusing on constructing a single summary measure of quality of life, statistical systems should provide the data required for computing various aggregate measures according to the particular perspective of each user.

The ideal measures of wellbeing – whether subjective, objective or mixed – are those that have the characteristics of validity and reliability/reproducibility, and which use as high a metric scale as possible.

At the time of writing, there is no single agreed metric used within central or local government. The aim must be to identify such a metric and ensure its consistent use. It is probably more important to the cause of wellbeing to obtain broad agreement to a metric that is adequate than to strive for the best possible measure:

> Because it is so hard to measure what is really important, governments and institutions pin down something else. But the consequences of pinning down the wrong thing are severe: all your resources will be focussed on achieving something you didn't mean to (Boyle, 2001: 45).

Established measures of wellbeing

In the early 1970s, economists James Tobin and William Nordhaus argued that gross national product (GNP), and a country's economic growth in general, was not a realistic measure of wellbeing, so they proposed a measure of economic welfare (MEW) that added other indicators to the GNP measurement (Nordhaus and Tobin, 1972). MEW adds the value of household services and leisure, and subtracts the cost of capital consumption, as well as pollution (Nordhaus and Tobin 1972: 513). Others have built upon this work, albeit using different weights for each scale.

The Index of Economic Wellbeing (IEWB), devised by the Canadian Centre for the Study of Living Standards (CSLS), includes physical and human capital as well as inequality, divorce rates and employment rates (CSLS, 1998). One of the most well-known measures of human living conditions is the UN's Human Development Index (HDI). It combines GDP with levels of life expectancy and education. The Weighted Index of Social Progress (WISP) is considerably more detailed, and includes forty social indicators such as education, health, status, gender equality, military expenditure, economy (including employment and income distribution), demography, environment, social chaos (political rights, corruption, war victims, refugees), cultural diversity and welfare effort.

Gross National Happiness (GNH) was devised by Bhutan's King Wangchuk in 1972 in order to reflect a more holistic approach to measuring the country's progress. The four pillars of GNH are the promotion of equitable and sustainable socio-economic development, preservation and promotion of cultural values, conservation of the natural environment, and establishment of good governance (Brooks, 2008).

A different approach is adopted in the Short Form (SF-36) (Ware *et al.*, 2008), which is a multipurpose health survey comprising 36 questions. The SF-36 provides, among other indices, psychometrically-based physical and mental health summary measures. The mental health component is a generic measure with four elements, vitality, social functioning, role, and emotional and mental health. The SF-36 has proven useful in surveys of general and specific populations, comparing the relative burden of diseases, and in differentiating the health benefits produced by a wide range of different treatments. It has been used in the International Quality of Life Assessment (IQOLA) Project.

Table 2.3 shows the SF-36 mental health component scores for the local authority areas in Wales in 2008. Of the two components of the SF-36 score, the mental health component is considered to measure more accurately the

Table 2.3   SF-36 mental component summary score

Mean	*Observed**			*Age-standardised**	
					*Unweighted base**
	Male	*Female*	*Person*	*Person*	
Local authority					
Isle of Anglesey	52.2	50.5	51.3	51.2	*1.295*
Gwynedd	52.9	50.8	51.8	51.8	*1.138*
Conwy	51.4	49.6	50.5	50.3	*1.189*
Denbighshire	51.2	49.8	50.5	50.5	*1.181*
Flintshire	52.0	50.0	51.0	51.0	*1.278*
Wrexham	51.3	49.4	50.3	50.4	*1.124*
Powys	52.3	49.5	50.9	50.9	*1.437*
Ceredigion	51.6	50.0	51.2	51.1	*1.470*
Pembrokeshire	52.3	59.2	51.2	51.2	*1.341*
Carmarthenshire	50.8	48.5	49.6	49.7	*1.268*
Swansea	51.0	48.2	49.6	49.5	*1.576*
Neath Port Talbot	50.4	47.7	49.0	48.9	*1.321*
Bridgend	50.7	47.4	49.0	49.0	*1.290*
The Vale of Glamorgan	51.4	49.3	50.3	50.4	*1.332*
Cardiff	50.0	48.2	49.1	49.2	*2.053*
Rhondda, Cynon, Taff	48.9	46.3	47.6	47.6	*1.645*
Merthyr Tydfil	49.1	45.7	47.3	47.3	*1.156*
Caerphilly	50.3	46.5	46.4	46.4	*1.282*
Blaenau Gwent	49.4	46.0	47.6	47.5	*1.207*
Torfaen	49.2	47.8	48.5	48.5	*1.253*
Monmouthshire	52.3	50.1	51.2	51.2	*1.551*
Newport	51.6	48.5	50.0	50.0	*1.170*
Wales	50.9	48.6	49.7	49.7	*29.557*

* Higher score means better health.

Source: Welsh Health Survey 2008.

mental state that is SWB. Of the local authority areas, Merthyr Tydfil (with an age-standardized mental health component score of 47.3) has the lowest level of wellbeing and Gwynedd (with an equivalent score of 51.8) the highest.

The SF-36 has been psychometrically tested in large UK samples with excellent response rates of around 70 per cent, satisfactory coefficients of reliability and validity, and responsiveness. Other practical considerations for its use include ease of administering the instrument and scoring, and the fact that it is so widely used. However, this instrument only measures short term, here and now wellbeing (W1).

Indices of Multiple Deprivation identify areas of multiple deprivation at the small geographical area level. Thus, they measure what can be conceptualized as the obverse or reciprocal of wellbeing. Each index is based on the fact that distinct dimensions of deprivation (such as income, employment, education and health) can be identified and measured separately. These dimensions, sometimes referred to as 'domains', are then aggregated to provide an overall measure of multiple deprivation, and each individual area is allocated a deprivation rank and score.

The latest version of the Welsh Index of Multiple Deprivation includes the following eight domains: income; employment; health; education, skills and training; housing; physical environment; geographical access to services; and community safety.

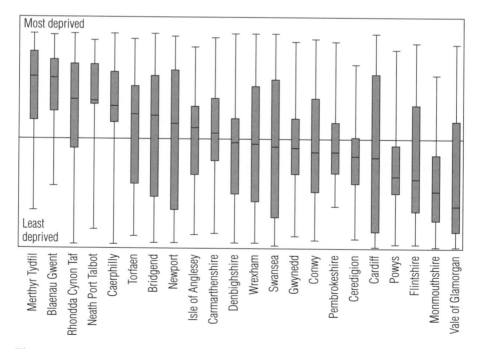

Figure 2.7   Overall level of deprivation for each local authority compared with the median ranks for Wales, 2005

Source: Welsh Assembly Government, Welsh Index of Multiple Deprivation 2005, Local Government Analysis. Reproduced under the Open Government Licence v.1.0.

Whether the weights applied to the various domain indicators to produce the overall Index are appropriate for measuring wellbeing is untested, so looking at the individual domain indices separately is probably more informative in indicating OWB.

Figure 2.7 displays the overall level of deprivation for each local authority in Wales in the year 2005 compared with the median All Wales level, and the distribution of deprivation scores within each local authority. The interpretation of this figure is that Merthyr Tydfil has the lowest wellbeing score in Wales and the Vale of Glamorgan the highest. Most commentators in Wales would agree that this accords with their own subjective qualitative assessment. The very large range of deprivation scores encountered in large conurbations (such as Cardiff) compared with the much narrower ranges found in the rural counties (such as Powys and Ceredigion) are noteworthy. The strong negative correlation between the deprivation measures and the SF-36 mental health component scores listed in Table 2.3 is as expected.

Evaluating policies, programmes and projects for wellbeing

Formal aids to the retrospective and prospective evaluation of policies, programmes and projects are not new. Financial accounting methods of various kinds were probably the first crude methods. It was rapidly realized, however, that simply looking at projects in terms of financial costs and benefits was not only inadequate, it failed to take account of the wider consequences on biodiversity and the environment, for example. In projects in developing countries, these were often substantial. This gave rise to environmental assessment alongside consideration of the financial costs and benefits.

In 1969, the USA introduced the Environment Protection Act 22, in the wake of Rachel Carson's book *Silent Spring*, which required an environmental impact assessment of all projects in the USA and all projects funded by US aid. This requirement was rapidly followed by other countries. Projects in developing countries were often associated with massive disruption of human communities, which could be displaced and have their culture and lifestyle radically changed. Despite this, often less attention was paid to the human species than to flora and other fauna! To correct this imbalance, social impact assessment was developed. The need to consider health issues in environmental impact assessment was also realized at an early stage.

Health impact assessment is closely allied to social impact assessment. The difference is one of emphasis and disciplinary mix, rather than one of substance. Both are concerned with impacts on human health and wellbeing. Recognition of the wide range of factors that determine health and the importance to health of non-health policy areas led to calls for healthy public policy and, by implication, the health assessment of policies. As Milio wrote in 1986 in her influential book *Promoting Health through Public Policy*, 'Health interests will be better served if the impact of policies affecting health, important aspects of environments and patterns of living were assessed.'

Considerable experience of health impact assessment in association with environmental impact assessment has been gained in Germany and in the

Netherlands. Much work was done in assessing the health impact of developments at Amsterdam's Schipol airport. The development of health impact assessment in the UK has been pioneered by public health specialists in Merseyside (Scott-Samuel, 1996): the first health impact assessment in which they were involved related to the proposed new runway at Manchester Airport.

Wellbeing impact assessment is merely a reformulation of health impact assessment, but it has the advantage of seemingly broadening its scope and its potential user audience by replacing the health yardstick with wellbeing.

Cost-utility analysis (CUA) is a form of economic analysis used to guide decisions where the outcome of a costed investment is measured in terms of its utility, rather than its financial consequences or attributes. So, in the field of health technology assessment (HTA), for example, the cost of investment is compared with health utility measured as quality adjusted life years (QALYs).

Cost wellbeing analysis is a form of cost utility analysis where wellbeing is the chosen utility measure.

Appraisal and evaluation in central government: the Green Book

Regulatory Impact Assessment (RIA), described in detail in HM Treasury's Green Book (2003), is now mandatory for all government programmes. In the White Paper, 'Choosing Health' in 2004, the UK government gave a commitment to build health into all future legislation by including health as a component in the Regulatory Impact Assessment.

The State of Happiness (Young Foundation, 2010) sums up the present position in terms of evaluating public policy:

> In the early 1990s when the current wave of interest in public policy and wellbeing started to gain momentum it was plausible to both say that happiness could not be measured and that it had little obvious relation to public policy. Neither position is tenable now. Happiness, wellbeing and fulfilment (all different things) are hard to measure but not inherently harder than GDP or educational levels. In a range of policy areas, many of which are highlighted in this report, there is plenty of evidence of correlation between policies and outcomes, and some evidence on causation.

(The use of the wellbeing framework for evaluating current drug policy in the UK is discussed in Chapter 10.)

Wellbeing as positive psychology/wellbeing promotion

Understanding wellbeing and its determinants not only enables policies, programmes and projects to be constructed and assessed according to their impact on wellbeing, it also allows a whole new community endeavour, analogous to health promotion: wellbeing promotion. This builds on the work of the Positive Psychology movement.

Wellbeing promotion is about empowering people acting on the conation element of the *eudaimonia*/wellbeing concept.

The Local Wellbeing Project – a partnership between the Young Foundation, Professor Richard Layard at the LSE, IdeA and three leading local authorities (Manchester City Council, South Tyneside Borough Council and Hertfordshire County Council) – began in 2006. The Project's aim was to find ways to accelerate local government's involvement in actions to increase wellbeing through practical trials and adapting mainstream services.

One of the elements the Local Wellbeing Project looked at was how practical initiatives within the three trial areas that aimed to improve community empowerment also contributed to resident wellbeing, and to develop an understanding of what could be done to strengthen this link.

The Young Foundation report, *Neighbourliness + Empowerment = Wellbeing* (Hothi *et al.*, 2008), drew on discussions with academics and experts, and with practitioners in the three areas. The report identified hypotheses from the evidence, in the UK and internationally, and tested them against case studies from the three local authority sites. It found that community empowerment contributes to resident wellbeing in three ways:

- by enhancing opportunities for residents to influence decisions affecting their neighbourhoods;
- by facilitating contact between neighbours and residents; and
- by helping residents to gain confidence to exercise control over local circumstances.

An interesting idea to come out of the first round of health, social care and wellbeing strategies in Wales was that of developing a community wellbeing axis. This would be based on the local general practice or health centre, working in partnership with other local institutions such as the local community college, which would both provide services relevant to wellbeing (such as advice on benefits and continuing education, respectively) and signpost others. Whether this idea is practicable when general practice seems to becoming more circumscribed and more focused under the new General Practitioner contract is debatable, but it could complement and strengthen the developing polyclinic model.

The New Economics Foundation, taking the 'five-a-day' mantra for dietary health as its model, has reviewed up-to-date evidence that suggests that building the following five actions into day-to-day lives is important for wellbeing:

- *Connect with the people around you*: With family, friends, colleagues and neighbours. At home, work, school or in your local community. Think of these as the cornerstones of your life and invest time in developing them. Building these connections will support and enrich you every day.
- *Be active*: Go for a walk or run. Step outside. Cycle. Play a game. Garden. Dance. Exercising makes you feel good. Most importantly, discover a physical activity you enjoy and that suits your level of mobility and fitness.

- *Take notice*: Be curious. Catch sight of the beautiful. Remark on the unusual. Notice the changing seasons. Savour the moment, whether you are walking to work, eating lunch or talking to friends. Be aware of the world around you and what you are feeling. Reflecting on your experiences will help you appreciate what matters to you.
- *Keep learning*: Try something new. Rediscover an old interest. Sign up for that course. Take on a different responsibility at work. Fix a bike. Learn to play an instrument or how to cook your favourite food. Set a challenge you will enjoy achieving. Learning new things will make you more confident as well as being fun.
- *Give*: Do something nice for a friend, or a stranger. Thank someone. Smile. Volunteer your time. Join a community group. Look out, as well as in. Seeing yourself, and your happiness, linked to the wider community can be incredibly rewarding and creates connections with the people around you.

In Wales, the Wellbeing Wales Network has been commissioned by the Welsh Assembly Government to develop, in conjunction with the New Economics Foundation, a Sustainable Wellbeing Assessment and Development Toolkit. The aim of this is to help organizations in all sectors to understand and enhance their wellbeing promoting role, and to provide a qualitative measuring framework against which to assess progress in improving local population sustainable wellbeing.

(The role of community development is wellbeing promotion, and the application of the toolkit is discussed in Chapter 8.)

Conclusion

The wellbeing notion has endured since ancient times because it seems to represent what most people would regard as what their lives, ideally, are about. A necessary refinement to the wellbeing concept that takes account of the growing concern with sustainable development is to add a forward-looking dimension to it, thereby constructing the concept of sustainable wellbeing.

To be useful in everyday life – rather than just in the annals of philosophers, psychologists and the like – wellbeing needs to be measurable. To this end, an ever-expanding armamentarium of measures has been developed over recent decades to permit the assessment of SWB and/or OWB.

These measures need to be applicable at different levels, ranging from the individual to neighbourhood, community, nation and globally. It is suggested that the SF-36 mental health component is such a measure of subjective short-term wellbeing (W1). For medium- and long-term wellbeing (W2 and W3), a single-item measure (such as the smiley/frowny face) linked to an appropriately worded long-term time frame question such as 'All things considered, how satisfied are you with your life as a whole so far?' is one option. One of the several available indices of multiple deprivation or equivalent measures would serve as measures of OWB. These are not ideal measures but are readily available, well-tested and, putatively, good enough for most probable uses.

To be able to measure human wellbeing is crucially important because, it is suggested, it is the unifying framework for all social policy and, as such, should be used by government at all levels to assess the impact of policies, programmes and projects. Techniques of impact assessment have been developed over the last fifty years, and these should be a mandatory and universal requirement of all actions undertaken in the public interest – not only to assess their overall impact on public wellbeing, but also to assess their impact on inequalities in wellbeing. We know from the work of Wilkinson and Pickett that reducing inequalities not only improves the wellbeing of the most disadvantaged, it also improves the wellbeing of all. Balancing impact on overall wellbeing against impact on inequalities in wellbeing will be a major challenge, as will balancing wellbeing impact today against its likely future impact.

As Ed Diener and Martin Seligman conclude in their monograph *Beyond Money: Toward an Economy of Wellbeing* (2004):

> Economic indicators have for the most part served society well. However, these indicators have glaring shortcomings as approximations, even first approximations, of wellbeing. Scientists are now in the position to assess wellbeing directly, and therefore should establish a system of national measures of wellbeing to supplement the economic measures. Indeed, it can be argued that the wellbeing measures should be the central ones, and that the economic indices are best understood in their relation to enhancing wellbeing. We have reviewed a number of important factors that influence wellbeing but are not captured by existing indicators, and we have shown the benefits of wellbeing in producing a successful society. It is time to grant wellbeing a prominent place in policy discussion.

Ways and means of promoting human wellbeing at individual and community levels also need to be developed, and the Positive Psychology movement, among others, offers ways of achieving this through mechanisms such as community development and the development of Wellbeing Centres.

(For further discussion of the implications of adopting the wellbeing framework as the universal yardstick of social progress and the driver of social policy, see Chapter 11.)

As Layard (2009: 92) has it:

> A good society is one where people are as happy as possible, and a few as possible are miserable. That is what many enlightened people believed in the eighteenth and nineteenth centuries. The time has come to reassert that humane philosophy and to put it into practice ... despite rapid rises in living standards, happiness has not risen over the past 50 years in Britain or the USA. If we want further rises in happiness, we need to focus seriously on what really causes happiness and misery.

For 'happiness' read 'wellbeing', which is 'happiness plus plus'.

Bibliography

Abdallah, S., Thompson, S., Michaelson, J., Marks, N., Steuer, N. *et al.* (2009) *The Happy Planet Index 2.0.* London: New Economics Foundation.

Andrews, F.M. and Withey, S.B. (1976) *Social Indicators of Well-being: Americans' Perceptions of Life Quality.* New York: Plenum Press.

Avineri, Shlomo (1968) *The Social and Political Thought of Karl Marx.* Cambridge: Cambridge University Press.

Bacon, N., Brophy, M., Mguni, N., Mulgan, G. and Shandro, A. (2010) *The State of Happiness: Can Public Policy Shape People's Wellbeing and Resilience?* London: Young Foundation.

Bailyn, Bernard (1992 [1967]) *The Ideological Origins of the American Revolution*, expanded edn. Cambridge, MA: Harvard University Press. BBC (no date) From a poll undertaken for the BBC by GfK NOP during October 2005. Results available at http://news.bbc.co.uk/nol/shared/bsp/hi/pdfs/29_03_06_happiness_gfkpoll.pdf.

Bentham, J. (1789) *An Introduction to the Principles of Morals and Legislation.* London: ch. 4.

Beveridge, W. (1942) *Report of the Inter-Departmental Committee on Social Insurance and Allied Services*, Cmnd 6404. London: HMSO

Boyle, D. (2001) *The Tyranny of Numbers: Why Counting Can't Make Us Happy.* London: HarperCollins.

Broadie, Sarah W. (1991) *Ethics with Aristotle.* Oxford: Oxford University Press.

Brooks, A. (2008) *Gross National Happiness: Why Happiness Matters for America – and How We Can Get More of It.* New York: Basic Books.

Carson, R. (1962) *Silent Spring.* New York: Houghton Mifflin.

Cooper, J.M. (ed.) (1997) *Complete Works*, by Plato Indianapolis: Hackett.

Cooper, Laurence (1999) *Rousseau, Nature and the Problem of the Good Life.* Pennsylvania: Pennsylvania State University Press.

Crosland, C.A.R. (1956). *The Future of Socialism.* New York: Macmillan.

Csikszentmihalyi, M (1990) *Flow: The Psychology of Optimal Experience.* New York: Harper & Row.

Department of Health (2010) 'Equity and Excellence: Liberating the NHS', Cmnd 7881.

Department of Health (1995) *Policy Appraisal and Health: A Guide from the Department of Health.* London: Department of Health.

Diener, E. (2009) *The Science of Well-Being.* New York: Springer.

Diener, E. (1984) 'Subjective Well-being', *Psychological Bulletin*, 95: 542–75.

Diener, E. and Seligman, M. (2004) 'Beyond Money: Toward an Economy of Wellbeing', *Psychological Science in the Public Interest*, 5: 11.

Doyle, W. (1981) *The Oxford History of the French Revolution.* Oxford: Clarendon Press. Easterlin, R. (1974) 'Does Economic Growth Improve the Human Lot? Some Empirical Evidence', University of Pennsylvania.

Epicurus (1998) 'Letter to Menoeceus, Principal Doctrines, and Vatican Sayings', in B. Inwood and L. Gerson, *Hellenistic Philosophy: Introductory Readings*, 2nd edn. Indianapolis: Hackett Publishing: 28–40.

Eurobarometer 69 (no date) available at http://ec.europa.eu/public_opinion/archives/eb/eb69/eb69_values_en.pdf.

Griffiths, S. and Reeves, R. (eds) (2009) *Well-Being. How to Lead the Good Life and What Government Should do to Help*, July. London: Social Market Foundation.

HM Treasury (2003) *The Green Book: Appraisal and Evaluation in Central Government.* London: TSO.

Hothi, M., Bacon, N., Brophy, M. and Mulgan, G. (2008) *Neighbourliness + Empowerment = Wellbeing: Is there a Formula for Happy Communities?* London: Young Foundation.

Howard, E. (1902 [1898]) *Garden Cities of Tomorrow.* Swan Sonnenschein & Co. Ltd.

Institute for Social and Economic Research (no date) *British Household Panel Survey*, Institute of Social and Economic Research, University of Essex.

Inwood, B. and Gerson, L. (1998) *Hellenistic Philosophy: Introductory Readings*, 2nd edn. Indianapolis: Hackett Publishing.

Johns, H. and Ormerod, P. (2007) 'Happiness, Economics and Public Policy', Institute of Economic Affairs, Research Paper 62.

Keane, J. (1995) *Tom Paine, A Political Life.* London: Bloomsbury.

Layard, R. (2009) 'Afterword', in Simon Griffiths and Richard Reeves (eds), *Well-being: How to Lead the Good Life and What Government Should do to Help.* London: Social Market Foundation. Local Government Act (2000) London: HMSO.

Maslow, A. (1970) *Motivation and Personality*, 2nd edn. New York: Harper & Row.

McGregor, J.A., Camfield, L., Masae, A. and Promphakping, B. (2008) 'Wellbeing, Development and Social Change in Thailand', *Thammasat Economic Journal*, 26(2): 1–27.

Milio, N. (1986) *Promoting Health through Public Policy.* Ottawa: Canadian Public Health Association.

Nettle, D. (2005) *Happiness: The Science behind Your Smile.* Oxford: Oxford University Press.

New Economics Foundation (2008) *Five Ways to Wellbeing.* London: New Economics Foundation.

NHS (2003) 'Health, Social Care and Well-being Strategies'. Cardiff: Welsh Assembly Government.

NHS (2002) 'Well Being in Wales'. Cardiff: Welsh Assembly Government.

Nietzsche, F. (2006 [1909]) *Thus Spoke Zarathustra*, Adrian del Caro (trans.) and Robert Pippin (ed.), Cambridge: Cambridge University Press.

Nordhaus, W. and Tobin, J. (1972) *Is Growth Obsolete?* New York: Columbia University Press.

OECD (2006) 'Alternative Measures of Well-being', OECD Statistics Brief 11, May.

Porter, R. (2000) *Enlightenment: Britain and the Creation of the Modern World.* London: Allen Lane.

Prescott-Allen, R. (2001) *The Wellbeing of Nations.* Canada's International Development Research Centre (IDRC) and Island Press, with the support of the IUCN and IIED.

Prime Minister's Strategy Unit (2002) 'Life Satisfaction: The State of Knowledge and Implications for Government', December, available at http://www.publications. parliament.uk/pa/cm200607/cmselect/cmpubadm/123/12311.htm.

Rose, G. (1992) *The Strategy of Preventive Medicine.* Oxford: Oxford University Press.

Scott-Samuel, A. (1996) 'Health Impact Assessment: An Idea Whose Time Has Come', *British Medical Journal*, 313: 183–4.

Seligman, M. (2003) 'Positive Psychology: Fundamental Assumptions', *Psychologist*: 126–7.

Sen, A. (1999) *Commodities and Capabilities.* Oxford: Oxford University Press.

Steuer, N. and Marks, N. (2008) *Local Wellbeing: Can We Measure It?* London: Young Foundation.

Stiglitz, J.E., Sen, A. and Fitousi, J.P. (2008) *Report by the Commission on the Measurement of Economic Performance and Social Progress.* Commission on the Measurement of Economic Performance and Social Progress.

Stout, A.K. (1967) 'Ross, William David', in P. Edwards (ed.), *The Encyclopaedia of Philosophy*. New York: Macmillan: 216–17.

UNICEF (2007) 'Child Poverty in Perspective: An Overview of Child Well-Being in Rich Countries', Innocenti Report Card 7. Florence: UNICEF Innocenti Research Centre.

Ware, J.E., Kosinski, M. and Dewey, J.E. (2001) How to Score – Version 2 of the SF-36 Health Survey (Standard & Acute Forms), 2nd edn. Lincoln, RI: QualityMetric Inc.

Welsh Assembly Government (2005) *Welsh Index of Multiple Deprivation* (WIMD). Welsh Assembly Government.

Welsh Office (1998) *Better Health, Better Wales*. Cardiff: Welsh Office.

Whitehall Wellbeing Working Group (no date) at http://www.defra.gov.uk/sustainable/government/what/priority/wellbeing/policy-context.htm.

Wilkinson, R. and Pickett, K. (2009) *The Spirit Level*. London: Allen Lane.

World Health Organization (1946) *Constitution*. Geneva: WHO.

Wellbeing: A Guiding Concept for Health Policy?

3

Marcus Longley

This chapter looks at the impact of the wellbeing concept on health policy and, in particular, on health care policy. It uses as a framework for analysis Robert Alford's social structures perspective and examines how each of the three structural interests – health care professionals, politicians and managers, and patients and the community – have reacted to the opportunities that the wellbeing concept ostensibly presents for policy development. It concludes by looking at some of the factors that would affect the adoption of the concept in the field of health and health care.

Introduction

Superficially, 'wellbeing' is an attractive concept for those concerned with health policy. Unsustainable growth in demand for health care, short-term public expenditure constraints, local community pressures and a growing intellectual curiosity about better ways of defining the purpose of public policy generally are all conducive to wellbeing as an organizing concept. But the chances of 'wellbeing' becoming a major theme in health policy depend on how the concept plays with the three key structural interests: politicians and managers, health professionals, and patients and the lay public.

For politicians and managers, there is a growing consensus about how health policy should be framed. They have moved beyond the old polarity of nanny state versus free market liberalism, to a 'non-ideological' recognition of the importance of both individual autonomy and the environment in which people live.

For many professionals, 'wellbeing' is a puzzling, subjective concept, difficult to apply to the urgent business of curing sick people. But new initiatives, such as patient reported outcome measures (PROMs), offer an early glimpse of how wellbeing might come to impact on their lives.

The concept of 'wellbeing' has ready appeal to lay people's common sense and is already evident, for example, in their patronage of complementary medicine. The ability to enlist lay enthusiasm for its application to the NHS could be a decisive factor in the future of the concept.

Peering beneath the surface of health policy

Trying to work out how health policy is developed and then implemented – or not – can easily give one a headache, and may not contribute to one's wellbeing. Why, for instance, are some policies repeatedly deemed a failure, yet others have miraculous success? Why are some goals a priority, and others not?

Since the 1970s, successive Secretaries of State for Health have proclaimed themselves disappointed by the lack of priority given to health promotion in the NHS, and have proceeded to launch a new initiative to achieve this goal ... only to be succeeded a few years later by the next Secretary of State, who similarly professes himself disappointed by the lack of progress ... and so on. But, on the other hand, the NHS struggled with waiting lists for decades and yet, within a few years at the start of the 2000s, these were all but abolished.

There seems to be either a variety of subterranean obstacles, or facilitators of health policy that mysteriously put goals on the table or take them off, and then water-down, undermine, or simply delay implementation. Some of the explanation probably has to do with competence – some policies were not much good – but there appears to be more to it than that.

One helpful approach to this perpetual conundrum is to think about how health services work (the NHS, and all those other elements that contribute to health), and who exercises power on and within them. In the early 1970s, the American sociologist Robert R. Alford was trying to work out why attempts to reform health care in New York City were failing. He used the lens of *social structures* to understand what was going on (Alford, 1975). Social structures are the social, political, legal, economic, cultural beliefs and institutions, and the relationships between them (especially structures of power), that make society function – constraining people, yet giving them the means of acting with apparent freedom. Each social structure has its own *structural interest*, a stake in something that is important to the structural interest because of the benefit or harm that it can do that particular interest group.

He identified three such structural interests in New York health care:

- clinicians, especially doctors, seeking clinical autonomy and interested in individual patients – these, he felt, were *dominant*;
- corporate rationalizers, a diverse group of government officials, managers, public health doctors, deans of medical schools and others who were concerned with populations of patients and the cost-effective use of resources – they were *challenging*; and

- patients and the community, whose interests were *repressed* by the other two groups.

Other scholars have subsequently applied this concept to UK health care, and have charted the rise of the challenging corporate rationalizers to a point (somewhere in the 1990s) where they have themselves become dominant, and are challenged by the clinicians (Harrison and McDonald, 2008). The patients and the community remained repressed, although arguably the thrust of health policy during the 2000s (in England, at least) has been to encourage a challenge from this structural interest, too.

This chapter uses Alford's insight to explore how the concept of wellbeing might fare in the UK health policy arena. What might it mean to the three key structural interests? In our contemporary context, they are re-defined as:

- *dominant*: governments, and their (semi-autonomous) agents, the managers of various sorts in the NHS and other bodies;
- *challenging*: clinicians, primarily doctors, but also nurses, allied health professionals and others; and
- *challenging*: patients, service users, their carers and communities (both geographical, and communities of interest).

Wellbeing, politicians and managers

At one level, of course, it is a gross over-simplification to think of all politicians and all managers as a single entity. What about differing political ideologies? What about all the different varieties of manager? However, there is a set of pressures that applies equally to all health ministers and the managers who work for them – budgetary constraints, patient and public expectations and tolerances, professional cultures within health care, and so on. These combine significantly to restrict freedom of movement for ministers and managers. And, in recent years, there has been a growing homogenization of ideology, as ministers become increasingly focused on 'managing' the services, and managers themselves increasingly emphasize the commonality between managing health care and any other service industry.

Early in 2010, the English Department of Health published a set of three 'Independent Reports', which they had commissioned from thinkers and practitioners outside the Department (Bernstein *et al.*, 2010; Mulgan, 2010; Reeves, 2010). Together, they provide an interesting encapsulation of 13 years of New Labour policy; they also fit quite comfortably with the broad approach of the new Conservative/Liberal Democrat administration. The fit with the three devolved nations may not be quite so comfortable: this will be looked at later.

At the time of writing, Richard Reeves is Director of the think tank Demos. His paper is about the proper role of the state in promoting health and wellbeing, and he argues for a new balance between helping people to live lives conducive to health and wellbeing, and personal freedom:

> The difficult question is how far a government should intervene in the choices and behaviour of individuals in order to promote their own health ... Research conducted for this review shows that people want to be healthy, and welcome government help to help make healthy choices easier. But the majority of citizens – men and women, rich and poor, old and young – value their freedom to make their own decisions, even if those decisions are unhealthy. Good health is a key ingredient of a good life. But so is freedom (Reeves, 2010: 3):

The conclusion is that governments hitherto have leant too heavily on the 'nannying' side of this balance, and need now to think about how to place greater value on individual freedom, while not abandoning collective goals for wellbeing:

> Government ... needs to strike a different tone in its messages around health and behaviour, with greater weight placed on informed choice and individual capacity (Reeves, 2010: 6).

This is not an isolated obsession: there is a widespread concern among policy-makers (especially in England) that trying to infringe upon personal freedom to achieve collective goals (such as wellbeing) is not only morally wrong, it also does not work. One of the most influential contributions to this debate in recent years came from the Chicago academics Richard H. Thaler and Cass R. Sunstein, whose book *Nudge: Improving Decisions about Health, Wealth and Happiness* (Thaler and Sunstein, 2008) argues for a 'libertarian paternalism' very similar to that of Reeves (and many others). Drawing on the work of behavioural economists, they sketch out what they call 'choice architecture' that will 'nudge' people in the right direction and 'edit' choices, while entirely supporting their ability to choose otherwise. The approach seeks to 'pad the path of least resistance', expect error, give feedback, and structure incentives carefully.

Geoff Mulgan – another think tank director – continues the theme with a look at 'what works' in changing behaviour. His conclusion also seeks to strike a realistic balance between the individual and the environment:

> People don't smoke or drink too much because they are ignorant, stupid or perverse – rather, it is the combination of the enjoyment that they get from these things and wider social or other environmental factors that mean they find it hard to adopt healthier behaviours (Mulgan, 2010: 4).

The answer is deliberately pragmatic: what works is what works. The work on the importance of equality for health (and other social) outcomes is important here (Wilkinson and Pickett, 2010). If the growing body of evidence is to be believed, striving for greater equality in society will itself improve health and wellbeing. The key element in this new evidence is the suggestion that *everyone* in society benefits from greater equality, not just the disadvantaged.

Berstein, Cosford and Williams come from the world of implementation, in local government and the NHS. Their treatment of 'wellbeing' – like that of Reeves and Mulgan – is interesting, in that they almost always link it to health: 'health and wellbeing' are almost inseparable. The intention here is to emphasize the fullness of the definition of health: certainly more than simply the absence of medically defined symptoms. And their practical message follows from this: public health and wellbeing should now concentrate not on extending life but, rather, on improving the quality of life. This is to be achieved by aligning national and local priorities to focus on *quality* and not *duration* of life; by better cross-government working, greater unity of purpose locally and a single inspection regime; by greater integration of the workforce (especially for children); and by a new vision of general practice.

Taken as a suite, these documents capture the zeitgeist. We have moved beyond nanny state *versus* free market liberalism, to a 'realistic' recognition of the importance of both individual autonomy and the environment in which people live; and, from this, follows a determination to develop ways of influencing people's wellbeing that respect such a synthesis, and which, therefore, actually work. An end to ideology; an embrace for empiricism. Given the dominant position of the political/managerial structural interest, this consensus is important, not only defining 'wellbeing', but also clarifying the parameters for its achievement.

Wellbeing and the professionals

The power of the health care professions to shape health policy in the UK has declined since the 1990s – perhaps with the exception of Scotland (Greer, 2004). They have moved from dominant to challenging, in Alford's terminology (Harrison and McDonald, 2008).

For more than 150 years, the power of the medical profession (followed much more recently by others such as nursing and midwifery) has been consolidated at three levels:

- Nationally, bodies such as the General Medical Council and the medical Royal Colleges have been afforded considerable formal and informal control over both their own profession and, by extension, over health care itself.
- At the institutional level, individual doctors have been given positions of considerable power as of right in NHS Trusts and other bodies. The existence of a post called 'Medical Director', testifies to this. (Since 2009, Local Health Boards in Wales now all have a Director of Therapies and Health Sciences to complement the Nursing and Medical Directors – so every clinician now has a direct route to the board.)
- At the individual patient level, there are a variety of formal and informal mechanisms that buttress the power of the doctor – from the exclusive legal power to prescribe drugs or certify sickness absence from work, to the ability to decide on the length of a consultation.

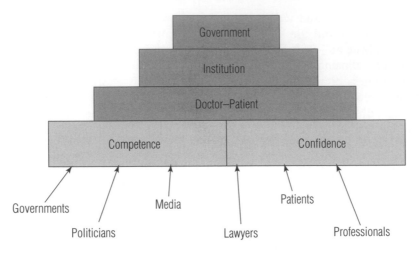

Figure 3.1   The eroding power of the professions

All of this power was historically built on two foundations: a general belief in the unique *competence* of doctors (only doctors could regulate doctors), and *confidence* that they would act in the interests of their patients. Both of these have been eroded over the last two decades by a combination of scandals and general scepticism about the position of all professions in society (see Figure 3.1)

This, in Alford's terms, marks the transition from 'dominant' to 'challenging'. To some extent, therefore, the views of the professions on wellbeing are irrelevant: they are no longer the dominant structural interest. But only to a certain extent ... the professions are by no means impotent; and wellbeing, if it has any currency, will be co-opted as a weapon in the ongoing struggle for dominance.

For many scientific rationalists (a key part of the paradigm of twenty-first-century medicine), wellbeing is a puzzling concept. What use is such a subjective notion? Even if it has some objective existence, where are the causal mechanisms that connect it to measurable morbidity and mortality? For many, the response to wellbeing is to discount it until/if such difficulties can be remedied. In the meantime, there are *really* sick people to cure. And, in the unfortunate event that managers or others might try to insist that wellbeing impinges much more on their 'clinical freedom', there is the time-honoured response of shroud waving: if you don't let me get on and do what I know best, people will die.

This will play differently as between *individual* clinicians – and also, to some extent, between different sub-specialties – and different health professions. Those that are more aware of the inter-relatedness between mind and body, and between individual and social context, may give greater credence to wellbeing, because they *know* that people do not get better and cope with their condition simply through a bio-medical fix such as surgery or pharmacotherapy. Such views may be bolstered or marginalized by the various organizations (themselves often closely allied to the political/managerial interest) that impinge on professional practice (such as NICE or the medical Royal Colleges) and, to some extent, by the individual or collective voices of patients.

The direct impact of the dominant structural interests is perhaps most effectively exercised through financial mechanisms within the NHS. The development of PROMs in England is one interesting development in this context:

> PROMs are measures of a patient's health status or health-related quality of life. They are typically short, self-completed questionnaires, which measure the patients' health status or health related quality of life at a single point in time. The health status information collected from patients by way of PROMs questionnaires before and after an intervention provides an indication of the outcomes or quality of care delivered to NHS Patients (Information Centre for Health and Social Care).

They were introduced for four specific procedures (hip replacement, knee replacement, hernias and varicose veins), and the use of questionnaires provides little scope for altering the pre-determined measurements. Nevertheless, they perhaps represent a significant shift towards systematically measuring the outcomes of NHS intervention over a longer period than has been usual; and also in regard to what matters in the context of a patient's life, not just in terms of the intentions of the surgeon. Ultimately, they might provide a set of metrics to assess whether the NHS is actually contributing to people's (self-defined) wellbeing. However, PROMs are still in their infancy, and it is difficult to see other ways in which 'wellbeing' might represent an immediate threat to professional power. This is, in part, because of the intrinsic difficulties in defining and measuring wellbeing set out in Chapter 1; it may also be because the measure has yet to fire the imagination of the other challenging interest: the patient and public. So, the sceptics can afford to ignore it, for the time being.

Wellbeing and citizens

It is something of a paradox that wellbeing has not yet captured the lay imagination. It does, after all, have its roots in people's lived experience, and is a 'commonsense' notion, in that it appeals to the sense of us all.

There is a plausible link between wellbeing and one area of people's health-seeking behaviour: complementary medicine. The growth of complementary medicine has been one of the fascinating aspects of health care over the past few decades. The concept is older than scientific medicine, of course, and is, at one level, the modern manifestation of the age-old human desire to seek comfort and hope against life's adversities wherever it can be found. To some extent, complementary medicine has been co-opted by governments and managers – for instance, by extending the regulatory regime for health care professionals to some of the complementary professions; and with a marginal incorporation of some techniques (such as acupuncture) into the NHS itself.

But complementary medicine remains largely outside the tax-funded sphere of health care in the UK, with chiropractors, osteopaths and others setting up their own premises in the high streets of most UK towns. This makes the recent growth of complementary medicine an even more eloquent testimony to people's desire for something more than conventional health care can provide: they have to pay for complementary treatments themselves. Some have argued that most of the attraction simply comes from spending more time with the complementary practitioner than the NHS can provide; others, that it is a cynical exploitation of people's desperation. There can, however, be little doubt of the popularity of complementary therapies, as people pay for what they perceive as effective treatment, often allied to a 'holistic' focus on the patient and their life. Some people, at least, are defining wellbeing by the services for which they are prepared to pay.

Another way in which patients can inject different nuances into the experience of health care is by campaigning and demanding something different from the NHS itself. Many observers have detected what they call a 'patient movement':

> Radical patient activists unpick part of the tapestry woven by more powerful, dominant social groups and try to weave a new pattern into it (Williamson, 2010: 4)

The aim of many is to change the way health care goes about its business, in order to improve most aspects of that business, including the wellbeing of the patient. The novelist P.D. James, who worked as a hospital administrator for many years, spoke for many when she wrote:

> To become a patient was to relinquish a part of oneself, to be received into a system, which, however benign, subtly robbed one of initiative, almost of will (James, 2008: 11)

It would appear that the NHS, while focusing on accurate and optimal diagnosis and treatment, does not always deliver care that supports and enhances people's wellbeing. Even 'insiders' – such as surgeon and erstwhile government Minister Lord Darzi – can be shocked by the inability of the caring service to care. He told *The Times* newspaper in 2008:

> What upsets me most is when the public are saying 'what we need is respect and dignity'. If we are not doing that, what the hell are we doing? (quoted in Williamson, 2010: 109).

There is a potentially powerful alliance to be struck between patients and the public, and whichever of the other two structural interests work out how to do the deal. Patients are increasingly clear about what they want from the NHS, and the missing element is often their broader wellbeing. Individual clinicians, clinical teams and whole professions are trying to work out how to deliver this, as are governments, managers and civil servants. Part of the deal is to establish measures of performance that assess patient wellbeing, and PROMs may be a part of this.

A much bigger challenge for them all is to overcome the NHS's 'institutional indifference'. The phrase 'institutional racism' was coined by Sir William Macpherson of Cluny in his 1999 report into the death of Stephen Lawrence. He found that the failure of the Metropolitan Police to conduct a competent investigation into Lawrence's murder showed that it was institutionally racist, which he defined as:

> The collective failure of an organization to provide an appropriate and professional service ... through unwitting prejudice, ignorance, thoughtlessness (*The Stephen Lawrence Inquiry: Report of an Inquiry by Sir William Macpherson of Cluny*, 1999).

The NHS appears unable to ensure that all its patients attain the feeling of dignity and receive the respect necessary for their wellbeing, although this is not through deliberate negligence, lack of resources or ill will. The term 'institutional indifference' appears appropriate.

Devolution within the UK

Whilst the suite of English Department of Health papers described earlier may reflect the élite English zeitgeist, the public discourse is rather different elsewhere in Great Britain, where centre-left parties of an older mould still hold sway. The political rhetoric conveys this different mindset. Take these phrases from the 2007 coalition agreement between Labour and Plaid Cymru in Wales:

> We are proud of the National Health Service, born in Wales ... We remain loyal and committed to these fundamental principles.

> We firmly reject the privatisation of NHS services or the organization of such services on market models.

> We are passionate about delivering significant improvements in the health of all of the people of Wales.

There is little evidence here of a new approach to the fundamental task of shifting people's behaviour. Rather, policymakers continue with an unquestioning belief in an older mix of exhortation, legislation and the power of communities and economic development to make a sufficient difference.

The term 'wellbeing', though, has considerable currency in the devolved nations. Wales, for example, has had 'health, social care and wellbeing' strategies since 2004. This tripartite approach, set within the context of overarching 'community plans', commands general support as a concept, with widespread acceptance of the need for joined up planning by all those agencies and sectors that can contribute to the population's wellbeing. There is considerable doubt, however, about the extent to which this really drives local developments – and resources allocation, in particular.

This pattern will continue to evolve – devolution is a process not an event – as a result of a series of objective pressures and subjective choices. The former will include shared demographic and epidemiological challenges across all four home nations, and a relatively common set of economic and fiscal challenges and opportunities. The dominant attitude towards wellbeing will be shaped by differences in the legal framework – each country currently has plans for small changes in the legislative framework affecting aspects of wellbeing that, in aggregate, start to assume significance as time goes by. There is also considerable experimentation taking place well away from the grand think tanks and policy elites, as local leaders explore new ways of delivering services and change policy 'from the bottom up':

> Policy is being made as it is being administered and administered as it is being made (Anderson, 1975: 98).

Devolution increases the scope for this variation. However, it is likely that any sustained changes at the local level will still conform to that country's dominant approach to health policy in general – and wellbeing, in particular.

Conclusion

At first sight, it is difficult to see how wellbeing might be a guiding concept for health policy. Policy on health has, in reality, been almost synonymous with policy on the NHS which, in turn, focuses on issues such as process success (waiting times), safety (avoiding scandals), resource management (balancing the books) and avoiding unnecessary obvious suffering (providing the latest treatments). The connection between these preoccupations and wellbeing is tenuous. Even those devolved nations, such as Wales, that tried to raise the policy gaze to the horizon and look at health gain, succumbed to the inevitable, as high waiting times forced people to look back at the problems at their feet.

But the context for health policy is changing. The growing pressure to address an unsustainable growth in demand for health care, short-term public expenditure constraints, local community pressures and a growing intellectual curiosity about better ways of defining the purpose of public policy generally are all conducive to a new look at wellbeing. Wellbeing offers ways out of all these dilemmas. It reframes the demand for more health care by asking, 'Is the marginal benefit worth having?' It can contribute to greater efficiency in the short term by bolstering the demand for the co-production of health, rather than the expectation that clinicians will provide, and people will consume health care. And it plays to a growing sense of community by highlighting the links between strong communities, social capital and wellbeing.

Achieving the incorporation of a new concept such as this into health policy is difficult since, in the process, it becomes the plaything of the competing structural interests. Ultimately, the power of this new currency will depend upon the robustness of the concept of wellbeing itself, and its measurability.

Bibliography

Alford, R.R. (1975) *Health Care Politics: Ideological and Interest Group Barriers to Reform*. Chicago: University of Chicago Press

Anderson, J.E. (1975) *Public Policy-Making*. New York: Holt, Praeger.

Bernstein, H., Cosford, P. and Williams, A. (2010) *Enabling Effective Delivery of Health and Wellbeing*. London: Department of Health.

Greer, S.L. (2004) *Territorial Politics and Health Policy: UK Health Policy in Comparative Perspective*. Manchester: Manchester University Press.

Harrison, S. and McDonald, R. (2008) *The Politics of Healthcare in Britain*. London: Sage.

Information Centre for Health and Social Care (no date) Available at http://www.ic.nhs.uk/proms (accessed 12 October 2010).

James, P.D. (2008) *The Private Patient*. London: Faber & Faber.

Mulgan, G. (2010) *Influencing Public Behaviour to Improve Health and Wellbeing*. London: Department of Health.

Reeves, R. (2010) *A Liberal Dose? Health and Wellbeing: The Role of the State*. London: Department of Health.

The Stephen Lawrence Inquiry: Report of an Inquiry by Sir William Macpherson of Cluny, Cm 4261, 1999.

Thaler, R.H. and Sunstein, C.R. (2008) *Nudge: Improving Decisions about Health, Wealth and Happiness*. New Haven and London: Yale University Press.

Wilkinson, R. and Pickett, K. (2010) *The Spirit Level: Why Equality is Better for Everyone*. London: Penguin.

Williamson, C. (2010) *Towards the Emancipation of Patients. Patients' Experiences and the Patient Movement*. Bristol: Policy Press.

Wellbeing and Spatial Planning

Alan Joyner

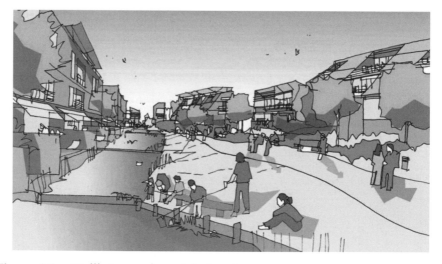

Figure 4.1   Wellbeing and spatial planning

Reproduced courtesy of Gallagher Estates.

This chapter examines what the promotion of wellbeing can mean as a concept for spatial planning if it is placed at the centre of local government activity as an inspiring ambition and ultimate policy objective.

Introduction

The pursuit of wellbeing and the practice of spatial planning for the physical environment are inextricably linked. A high standard of wellbeing and good quality of life can be influenced by the policies adopted by a local authority and the delivery of its services.

Sustainable development is central to the UK planning system and closely allied to wellbeing. The history of public health and town planning contains valuable lessons that can be drawn upon to influence the future policies of local authorities and the delivery of local services.

Rapid large scale social, economic and environmental changes, together with the impact of political change, will affect people's future wellbeing. More cost-effective, economic and efficient ways of future working by local authorities will be crucial, if satisfactory standards of front line services are to be maintained.

Partnership working between local authorities and other agencies – public bodies, the private sector and the voluntary sector – will be an increasingly important aspect of service delivery. A high standard of wellbeing and quality of life through improved performance and effective partnerships is a worthwhile objective for local government.

The promotion of wellbeing needs to be part of a continuing process involving a vision, a methodology for assessing and measuring the outcome, and collaborative initiatives to deliver and review what has been achieved. Community-based initiatives – in which local people have a greater say over how money is spent and have the right to control and be involved in running local facilities – will assume greater importance because of policy changes that are driving this political agenda.

Wellbeing and the physical environment

What sort of life do people want to lead; and what do they want from their lives, for themselves and their communities? Can a high standard of happiness and wellbeing, and a good quality of life be attained through appropriate policies and effective delivery of local services? A detailed definition of wellbeing and its meaning, origins and development is given in Chapter 2 and is not within the scope of this chapter. There is considerable ambiguity and conceptual diversity around the definition, usage and function of wellbeing (Ereaut and Whiting, 2008: 1) which, on analysis, turns out to be a multi-dimensional state comprising objective criteria and subjective feelings.

Almost every planning decision or policy has a potential effect on mental and physical wellbeing. It is widely acknowledged that the spatial planning of the urban and rural environment plays an important role in determining the quality of life within communities. Sustainable patterns of development, the protection and creation of good quality sustainable environments and the provision of access to employment, housing and other facilities (such as those for health, education, open space, sport, recreation and transport) all contribute to good health and wellbeing. Effective local government has wide-ranging concern for the wellbeing of its population and an extensive range of powers available to take appropriate action.

The rapid pace of change affecting wellbeing in social, economic, environmental and political terms is on a large scale, including the significant impact of climate change. How effectively these changes are tackled will determine their future impact on wellbeing associated with the physical environment. The immediate future economic prospect is one of austerity due to imposed public spending reductions which will affect the ways in which government departments, local authorities and other agencies will be able to respond.

There are more fundamental questions:

- Is the pursuit of a high standard of wellbeing entirely dependent on an increasing level of material income and wealth where there are large inequalities within society?
- Is this compatible with the principle of sustainable economic growth that can be sustained within environmental limits whilst enhancing environmental and social welfare?
- Furthermore, is the pursuit of a high standard of wellbeing affordable, and can it survive future economic cycles?
- Is it worth examining whether wellbeing can be a central goal for the achievement of future healthy and contented communities, and a driving force and unifying framework for spatial planning?
- Is there scope for improving the joining up and integration of local services to achieve this aim and deliver a better quality of life?

Most important of all, is to consider the need for more effective and inclusive ways of securing community and individual involvement in local decision-making, and for giving local authorities more responsibility for formulation of policy and delivery of services at the local level. This is capable of being focused, with public support and engagement, around a principal objective of wellbeing making a real difference to the places where we live. Such action is consistent with the statutory duty of local authorities to promote understanding among local people of the opportunities that exist for them to get involved in, and influence, the decisions made by local authorities and other public bodies (Local Democracy, Economic Development and Construction Act 2009: ch. 1, s. 1)

The urban and rural environments, and how they are used and managed, have always been fundamental to human health and wellbeing. Many town planning public health decisions and wider public policies have an impact. The concept of sustainable development with social, economic and environmental considerations is central to the UK planning system, and can be closely allied to the concept of wellbeing.

Despite collaborative working between planning and public health professionals, the linkages have not always been well connected. Each branch of public policy is often pursued independently, thus failing to grasp the integrated nature of real life. For example, health authorities and public health programmes have provided services for those who are ill, for controlling communicable diseases and for dealing with drug addiction; whereas, planning authorities have been concerned principally with environmental protection and economic development, rather than health promotion. Spatial planning has a key role to play in tackling these problems; shaping the physical environment; and making it possible for people to make healthier choices about exercise, local services, travel, nutrition, taking an interest in nature and participation in leisure activities. It has been acknowledged that 'physical, mental and social wellbeing directly corresponds to the concept of sustainable communities synonymous with spatial planning' (RTPI, 2009: 4).

The former Labour government launched the Sustainable Communities Plan in February 2003, setting out a long-term programme of action for delivering sustainable communities in both urban and rural areas. The main aim was to deal with housing supply issues, and conceive a new approach to the quality of layout and design of residential areas and public open spaces within new communities in designated growth areas (Office of the Deputy Prime Minister, 2003).

In 2010, the Coalition government took a different view of how new communities and housing should be delivered, and believed that it was time for a fundamental shift of power from Westminster to people at the local level, and radical changes to the planning system. It intended to promote decentralization and democratic engagement, and to end the era of top-down government by giving new powers to local councils, communities, neighbourhoods and individuals (HM Government, Cabinet Office, 2010a: 11, s. 4). These principles were subsequently included in draft legislation (Localism Bill, 2010).

The promotion of wellbeing associated with greater community involvement is an opportunity for new and existing communities to improve inclusiveness and fairness, and reduce social inequalities to create sustainable patterns of development. There are new challenges. Health and wellbeing are key considerations in climate change and the danger that this poses. An increasing rate and scale of landscape change will occur, together with new patterns of recreation and tourism with more scope for recreational outdoor physical activities. The value of therapeutic landscapes to human health is an example of how the spatial environment matters to wellbeing (Healing Landscapes website, April 2011). Urban and rural development, if managed effectively with behavioural change and adaptation of existing places, will support a better standard of wellbeing, which will contribute to economic growth. A transition towards a low carbon transport system, renewable sources of energy, energy efficiency and more physical activity, among other measures, could reduce the impact of urban air pollution and climate change caused by carbon emissions (Defra, 2010: 4).

There will be higher standards for house building through the 'Code for Sustainable Homes', with a target of zero carbon homes by 2016 (DCLG, 2006a: 2). These former Labour government policy initiatives remained part of the Coalition government's agenda in 2011, and local authorities are expected to play their part in delivery. They will need to gear up to deliver their services in a challenging environment that will need to be joined up and integrated with those of other agencies to achieve the development of sustainable communities and a high standard of community wellbeing.

Although the word 'wellbeing' was introduced in the context of giving every local authority the power to promote the social, economic and environmental wellbeing of their area (Local Government Act 2000, pt 1, s. 2), the implications of this initiative seem, at times, not to have been fully understood. Debate has often been conceived solely in uni-dimensional departmental terms within strict professional boundaries, with no overall view of its purpose. At a time of public expenditure restraint, there is a need to be more efficient in delivering local services; local authorities will be expected to 'deliver more with less', and to promote the high standards of services and quality of life that are necessary to meet the needs of all sections of the community.

This could be the *raison d'être* for community action under the idea of 'Big Society' to reinvigorate local accountability, democracy and participation, which the Coalition government, in 2010d, put at the heart of public service reform (HM Government, Cabinet Office website, 2010b; DCLG, 2010).

Wellbeing, spatial planning and public health

The pursuit of wellbeing, joined with sustainability and spatial planning to establish a link between health and happiness, is not an entirely new concept. The origins of modern town planning emerged from the public health movement of the nineteenth century, which developed an understanding of the impact of poor housing, the environment and living conditions upon human health, wellbeing and happiness, and the need for change through the work of Edwin Chadwick and others (Chadwick, 1842). The landmark report by Friedrich Engels in 1844 gave a detailed description and analysis of the appalling conditions of the working classes, and is an important record of the relationship at that time between the environment, lack of spatial planning and the effect on wellbeing. The creation of Local Boards of Health by the Public Health Act 1848 led to the landmark Public Health Act 1875, with its raft of powers relating to public health and building byelaws. The Local Government Acts of 1888 and 1894 established the local authorities that were to become responsible for these functions.

Furthermore, there were literary influences in the nineteenth century, by the likes of Benjamin Ward Richardson – a physician, anaesthetist, physiologist and sanitarian (Richardson, 1876); James Hole – a reformer, educationalist and advocate for the erection of model villages outside large towns (Hole, 1866); and other contemporaries. They began to theorize about city life and urban form in the light of the prevalent wretched condition of many industrial towns, and to make the links between public health, housing and planned developments. The industrial reformers followed with the first positive steps towards developing new communities, often from a mixture of self-interest and moralistic idealism. An early example was the new model community at Saltaire built by Titus Salt in 1850 (James, 2004): he moved his mill out of Bradford to a new site where he provided community facilities, open space, parks, churches, almshouses, public baths and washhouses. Another was Bourneville village built in 1893 on the outskirts of Birmingham by Richard and George Cadbury. The object was to provide facilities alongside their new factory where workers could live in far better conditions than in the crowded slums of the city. The facilities included houses with ample gardens, open space and playgrounds (Harvey, 1906). The improvement in the environment and spatial planning of these developments was a great stride forward. However, the political and moral nature of these new planned communities should also be recognized, as they were promoted under a moralizing agenda with religious underpinning. Titus Salt was active in politics and was Mayor of Bradford in 1848. The Cadbury Family were Quakers.

The influence of the garden city concept and new towns movement in the history of British town planning cannot be underestimated. At the turn of the twentieth century, Ebenezer Howard read widely and thought deeply about social issues, and published his proposal for the creation of new towns of limited size, planned in advance and surrounded by a permanent belt of agricultural land. There can be no doubt of Howard's understanding of the attainments of health, wellbeing and happiness through access to green spaces and the countryside (Howard, 1898). He developed these ideas into the garden city concept and the new towns movement (Howard, 1902). Figure 4.2 illustrates

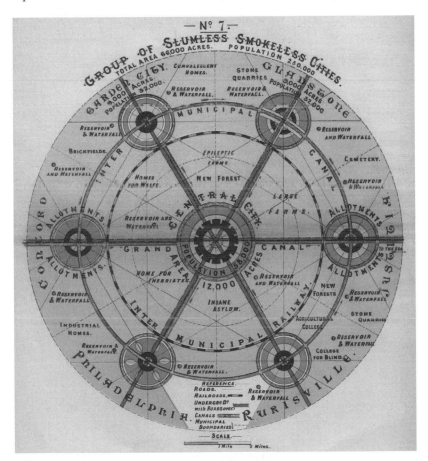

Figure 4.2   Howard's ideal plan for a cluster of garden cities

Source: Howard (1898), reproduced courtesy of the Town and Country Planning Association.

Howard's ideal plan for a cluster of garden cities against a green backcloth, located around a larger central city and linked by transport corridors through a surrounding agricultural belt. Housing was to be located in a clean environment away from the industrial zone, with tree-lined avenues and boulevards separating the zones. In the centre, was to be an ornamental garden surrounded by the main public buildings and a park, shops and exhibitions.

Letchworth in Hertfordshire was the first garden city, designed by Ebenezer Howard in 1903. Today, the town represents many of the ideals that Howard strove for – a modern, clean town with a balance of residential houses, open space, shopping facilities and industrial areas. Welwyn Garden City was Howard's second new town, developed in 1920. The residential and industrial areas are laid out along tree-lined boulevards with a neo-Georgian town centre that offers excellent shopping facilities, open space and sports facilities. The design and planning of these two new towns provide good historic examples of the creation of environments that enhance wellbeing.

These ideas became part of British planning doctrine and practice that, following the beginning of town planning legislation in the twentieth century (including the New Towns Act of 1946 and the Town and Country Planning Act 1947), led to the creation of the first phase of postwar new towns beyond the London greenbelt. The New Towns programme is often referred to as one of the most ambitious urban planning exercises of the twentieth century. The new towns sought to address many wellbeing related issues, including housing shortages, economic growth and the creation of 'balanced communities' through mixed tenure housing and a range of industry.

More recent examples of new town building and urban extensions include Milton Keynes in Buckinghamshire and Poundbury in Dorset. Milton Keynes was formally designated on 23 January 1967, with a design brief to develop in size at the scale of a city. Milton Keynes Development Corporation planned the major road layout according to street hierarchy principles, using a grid pattern at one kilometre intervals, rather than on more conventional radial patterns. With a population currently of more than 200,000 and with 130,000 available jobs, the city is one of the UK's fastest growing urban areas; by 2031, it will be the 16th largest city in England (Invest Milton Keynes, 2007). Poundbury is the urban extension to Dorchester and has become cited as a pioneering example of urban development. It seeks to implement the town planning and design principles expounded by the Prince Charles (HRH The Prince of Wales, 1989) for exemplary environmental and sustainability standards. Poundbury is expected to be completed by 2025 with housing for approximately 5,000 and 2,000 available jobs.

There were criticisms of new towns that many were built on greenfield sites and, in the early years, the developments were seen as boring, with houses that lacked character and created a sense of isolation within the community. Early new towns failed to attract the intended 'social mix', with those near London having residents commuting at a higher level than was anticipated. It should be recognized that, notwithstanding the successful rapid growth of more recent new towns such as Milton Keynes, this is not the only consideration to the exclusion of other social and environmental issues. Poundbury also has its critics, because of its moralizing undertones. Lessons now being learnt from the new towns are being evaluated with the intention of identifying good practice and avoiding mistakes in the future planning of new communities (DCLG, 2006b).

Influential architects of the twentieth century also had an impact on spatial planning and design. Examples are Le Corbusier's theory for urban planning based on a high rise commercial centre, with parks and trees surrounded by geometrically designed residential areas and outer suburbs (Le Corbusier, 1987), and Lloyd Wright's ideas on the promotion of organic architecture, including original and innovative examples of many different building types, urban and suburban development concepts and his proposals for Broadacre City (Lloyd Wright, 1932).

Good architectural design for creating a physical environment that enhances wellbeing to a greater degree can promote high quality, sustainable and healthy places. The Commission for Architecture and the Built Environment advocates an all-inclusive approach to planning, building and managing places that affect people's health and wellbeing (CABE website, 2010). Planning legislation and practice was developed by concerning itself strictly with 'land use' matters, and no clear link, although implied, was explicitly established between planning, development and health until the statutory requirement was introduced for development plans to embrace the objective of contributing to the achievement of sustainable development (Planning and Compulsory Purchase Act (P&CP Act) 2004, pt 3, s. 39).

The spatial planning strategy, established through changes in national planning policy, provided for a new process involving the preparation of Local Development Frameworks containing a number of inter-related documents. The key aims of the former Labour government in this process were flexibility, strengthening community and stakeholder involvement, front loading by taking decisions early in the preparation of plans, sustainability appraisal, programme management and soundness in process and content based upon a robust, credible evidence base (P&CP Act 2004, pt 2, ss. 17–28).

This wider scope of spatial planning – taking account of the social, economic and environmental impacts of development – is akin to the same components of wellbeing contained in the Local Government Act 2000. This signalled an important change to planning in England and Wales, bringing in a new focus on spatial planning going well beyond traditional land use planning, and it continues to provide an opportunity for the concept of wellbeing to take centre stage. Spatial planning was to have an emphasis on improved coordination and consultation. More recent legislation (Local Democracy, Economic Development and Construction Act, 2009) provided for a new regional planning regime centred on a single regional strategy covering housing, transport and economic development; this was to be developed jointly by the Regional Development Agencies (RDAs) in partnership with newly established Local Authority Leader's Boards.

The former Labour government intended these strategic plans to join up land use, planning and economic development (including transport and housing) with a vision for regional prosperity over a period of 15 to 20 years. This included a new requirement for councils to undertake an economic assessment of their area to understand the challenges, make informed decisions and contribute to the development of the regional strategy.

However, the political context changed. In 2010, the Coalition government published draft legislation (The Localism Bill, 2010) to abolish the legal basis for Regional Spatial Strategies, to devolve greater powers to councils and neighbourhoods, and to give local communities control over housing and planning decisions (Number 10 website, 2010). The Local Authority Leader's Boards were scrapped and the Coalition government reduced spending commitments in June 2010, with a saving of £16 million. (HM Treasury, 2010). In addition, a new economic model was introduced that included the creation of Local Enterprise Partnerships, for joint local authority-business bodies to promote local economic development and replace Regional Development Agencies (Department for Business Innovation and Skills, 2010). Regional Strategies were formally revoked in July 2010 (DCLG, 2010c). Further severe public spending reductions were announced in the government's Spending Review in October 2010. As a consequence, private and public sector funding will be in much shorter supply in the future.

Prior to the general election in May 2010, the Conservative Party published a Policy Green Paper, 'Open Source Planning', which heralded the intention to make radical changes to the planning system and to the Local Development Frameworks introduced by the former Labour government. New local plans are to be built out of a process of collaborative democracy (Conservative Party, 2010: 8)

The Coalition government promoted legislation in 2011 (Localism Bill) to give effect to these changes with a greater degree of involvement, participation and decision-making to be devolved to local councils and communities. It stressed the importance to be attached to local spatial plans. It linked its commitment to localism as a theme within reinvigorated spatial planning. A national planning framework was published in 2010, and radical changes in housing and planning are intended to drive local growth (HM Treasury and the Department for Business Innovation and Skills, 2011).

The wide scope of spatial planning fits easily with the concept of wellbeing as a champion for the pursuit of happiness, health and prosperity. Coupled with greater involvement and empowerment of local communities in the day-to-day decisions that affect their lives, wellbeing can become a driving force for the development of future public policy at local level.

The need to focus on key priorities, working to a clear framework with a joined-up approach and stakeholder involvement is an important objective at a time of financial restraint and public spending reductions. The pursuit of wellbeing can be central to this objective and can be delivered by local authorities working locally in partnership with other agencies.

Wellbeing and improving performance

Since the mid-1990s, it has become increasingly clear that wellbeing depends on a number of different factors that include personal genetic make-up, the neighbourhoods in which we live and grow up, lifestyle choices, employment, income, and access to services and facilities. Local authorities play a fundamental role in creating the environment for communities to prosper, and need to ensure that the impact on health and wellbeing is a positive one. In 1998, the former Labour government announced its programme to modernize local government based on the themes of community leadership, democratic renewal and improving performance in services (DETR, 1998: 12). Community leadership was to be promoted through powers of wellbeing, and a duty to undertake community planning and partnership working. Improved performance was to be achieved through the implementation of a modernization agenda for local government.

Democratic renewal was tackled through radical changes made by the Local Government Act 2000 (pt II), which provided for new political management structures for local authorities in England and Wales, including London Boroughs. The existing system of governance was replaced by new executive arrangements, which have made significant changes to the conduct of business.

The promotion of wellbeing as a beneficial concept for health and happiness offers a promising means by which to persuade a local authority to place it at the centre of policymaking for spatial planning and delivery of local services. In Scotland, improving wellbeing has been recognized as a top priority for local government, with incentives for creating healthy environments, strengthening community action, tackling health inequalities and working to develop partnerships (NHS, Health Scotland, 2007: 15). This has been achieved through 'joined up action' to enhance wellbeing through partnership and collaborative working.

Partnership in wellbeing and community planning

The concept of community is ill defined and ambiguous, and may be interpreted in a number of ways. Individuals may belong to more than one community based on place, identity or interest. Neighbourhood design and layout can facilitate community cohesion, interaction and integration, but social interaction, behaviour and active involvement by people in the use of these places is required to engender the sense of belonging and attachment that makes for a successful and sustainable community. Local authorities are central to bringing together all public sector organizations, the private sector, the community and voluntary sectors to ensure that there is a concerted and inclusive approach to improving community and individual wellbeing.

The concept of community leadership posits a role for local authorities being concerned for the wellbeing of the communities for which they provide services. It expects local authorities to respond to the needs and aspirations of their population and communities. The statutory power to promote wellbeing and to improve the quality of life of their communities is a clear responsibility (Local Government Act, 2000: s. 2), and they can improve their efficiency and effectiveness by joining up the delivery of services and using the wide-ranging powers of wellbeing that are now available. However, this is not always straightforward, as there is a multiplicity of organizations in an area whose activities need to be coordinated, including the strategic health authority, the health trusts, the primary care groups, sixth-form colleges, further and higher education institutions, the Learning and Skills Council, the police authority, joint boards for services such as fire and public transport, and housing associations, plus the many agencies of central government (Stewart, 2003: 14).

This led to the duty imposed on local authorities to prepare community strategies to engage and involve local communities, involve active participation of councillors, be based on a proper assessment of needs and availability of resources, and be prepared and implemented by a broad 'local strategic partnership' through which the local authority can work with other local bodies (DETR, 2000: 7).

Detailed guidance for developing and implementing the strategies included the stages of establishing a vision, establishing priorities and an action plan, and delivering community priorities; coordinating and rationalizing local activity; and monitoring and measuring progress, followed by a review process (DETR, 2000: 22–9).

Establishing a vision for a community strategy at the outset provides an opportunity to place wellbeing at the centre of the vision, and to advocate its beneficial credentials for attaining health and happiness for communities and individuals. However, considerable care is required, as a vision for 10 or 20 years ahead makes no allowance for the unforeseen changes that will take place in the future, or the uncertainties that lie in the present. As has been pointed out, a vision drawn up 20 years ago would not have taken account of the growth of the Internet or the extent of globalization (Stewart, 2003: 19). Thus, the process of community planning has to be a continuous process, continually analyzing existing problems and opportunities, monitoring outcomes of actions, considering future changes and what needs to be done to meet these.

The formation of a local strategic partnership as a single body for the process of community planning has been adopted by many local authorities. The idea is to bring together at a local level the public sector as well as the private, business and voluntary sectors to tackle a wide range of issues and initiatives, with participants working closely together to coordinate efforts and give mutual support (DCLG, 2010d). The Conservative Party's pre-election Planning Green Paper in 2010 called for greater public involvement and participation in public policy and decision-making, and advocated localized 'open source planning' through which communities are empowered over a much wider range of issues (Conservative Party, 2010). The use of the 'open source' idea, which flows out of information technology, appears to be based on much greater community involvement which, in turn, is referenced as 'collaborative democracy'. This is a strong commitment to bottom-up planning, with communities defining objectives and needs on a neighbourhood scale with individual plans bolted together to form a local plan. This forms part of the 'Big Society' approach of the Coalition government that was announced in 2010 (HM Government: Cabinet Office, 2010a).

The Coalition government intends to go further to encourage more community and individual involvement in decision-making by distributing power and opportunity to people, rather than within government (HM Government Cabinet Office, 2010b: 7). These ideas build on a long-standing perception of a disconnection between communities and the planning process, and include the difficult problem of integrating national imperatives and local aspirations. This is likely to cause problems for some in embracing public involvement, if it is intended to be influential, overriding, decisive and conclusive to all other considerations in decision-making.

There is recent evidence suggesting that public knowledge and interest in local government and local issues has fallen sharply in recent years. The findings were that the proportion of the public claiming to have a 'great deal' or a 'fair amount' of knowledge about their council had fallen to 40 per cent from 47 per cent over the course of three years. Actual knowledge of local government was even lower, with only 36 per cent of the public aware that the statement 'most of the money that local councils spend is raised locally, through council tax' is false. Only 19 per cent of respondents claimed to be 'very interested' in local issues, compared with 32% in per cent earlier surveys (Hansard Society, 2010). This is reinforced by the Citizenship Survey published in July 2010, which found that in 2009/10, only 37 per cent of people felt they could influence decisions in their local area (HM Government, 2010c).

This apparent reduction in the level of public interest and involvement in local government affairs has occurred notwithstanding the statutory 'Duty to Involve' introduced by the former Labour government in 2007 (Local Government and Public Involvement in Health Act, 2007, s. 138).

The current policy initiatives – for 'Localism' and 'Big Society', together with the statutory duties introduced by the former Labour government and recent evidence about the falling level of public interest – suggests that renewed efforts and incentives are required to undertake successful community planning, and to increase people's interest in public policymaking and seeking to influence decisions that affect the physical environment. The potential for wellbeing issues to drive this agenda is strong at a time when faced with future social, economic and environmental impacts arising from climate change, including increased greenhouse gas emissions causing atmospheric changes, increased temperature, rainfall and rising sea levels (Meteorological Office, 2009). To combat this, at a time of financial spending restraint and relative austerity due to the current national economic deficit, significant lifestyle changes will be needed.

The opportunity to organize and plan around a central theme of community and personal wellbeing is a compelling one. At the community level, there is the potential to coordinate and join up the delivery of services to the benefit of healthy and contented communities. At the personal level, there are the incentives of enjoying the advantages and satisfaction of a healthier lifestyle, and a better quality of physical environment and surroundings.

Measuring sustainable wellbeing

A high level of wellbeing is thought to be a feature of strong and vibrant communities; an individual's or community's wellbeing depends on many issues including:

(i)   people's interest and engagement in the community, and their sense of control over their own lives;
(ii)   happiness and feelings of confidence and self-esteem;
(iii)   being treated with dignity and respect;
(iv)   access to affordable nutritious food;
(v)   a sense of security – financial and otherwise;
(vi)   access to services, facilities and opportunities;
(vii)   the care and support that is available when needed;
(viii) comfort and overall quality of life;
(ix)   spiritual needs and respect for faith and religion;
(x)   access to affordable, safe, secure and appropriate housing;
(xi)   protection from crime and disorder; and
(xii)   people's work, home and recreational environments.

(Welsh Assembly Government, 2007: 5)

A mutually beneficial relationship between health, wellbeing and sustainability is apparent, and it is clear that their close relationships suggest it is wrong to consider them as separate concepts. Health is substantially affected by wellbeing and vice versa; without sustainability, both concepts are based on weak foundations. At the heart of any concept of wellbeing and sustainable development must be the ability to identify and quantify the trade-offs that exist between elements of an individual's and other people's current wellbeing and wellbeing in the future. How wellbeing will be conceptualized by policy-makers will ultimately turn on their normative judgements about the implications that follow from these various trade-offs (Dolan et al., 2006: 4).

The measurement of wellbeing is dealt with in some detail in Chapter 2, and it is beyond the scope of this chapter to consider anything other than that related to spatial planning and the physical environment. It cannot be fully measured by any single indicator. It seems clear that measuring wellbeing should be approached from two directions. First, as objective wellbeing or quality of life, it can be broken down into a number of key components. The former Dyfed Powys Health Authority model based on the Index of Multiple Deprivation continues to provide a platform on which to build (Dyfed Powys, 2002). Second, as subjective wellbeing or happiness/mental health, many measures have been proposed but probably nothing beats the simplest measure of all, the smiley faces 'emoticon' array, as commonly used in happiness research (Bond, 2003; Fahlman, no date).

The Department for the Environment Food and Rural Affairs (Defra) has published a list that combines existing sustainable development indicators, along with related supplementary wellbeing measures to cover life satisfaction. The wellbeing indicators and measures related to the physical environment include overall life satisfaction, positive and negative feelings, engagement in positive activities, local environment, feelings of safety, health and physical activity, green space, cultural participation and positive mental health (Defra Sustainable Development website).

The use of a 'Sustainability Assessment Framework' technique using integrated resource management modelling (IRM) to score key performance indicators against a range of sustainability objectives has been used recently in the planning of a proposed new community at Northstowe in Cambridgeshire (Arup, 2007). Figure 4.3 illustrates the technique, which is to divide the assessment into four quadrants – Environment, Social, Economic and Natural Resources. The quadrants are then subdivided into further segments, each representing one of the sustainability objectives. Behind each objective are key performance indicators by which the performance of each objective is measured.

Another analytical technique is Health Impact Assessment (HIA), which is increasingly being used to inform planning decisions for large, mixed-use developments (Department of Health, 2010) but a more informal, accessible and readily understood process would be preferable to encourage the interest and involvement of local communities in the further development of existing, new and expanded communities.

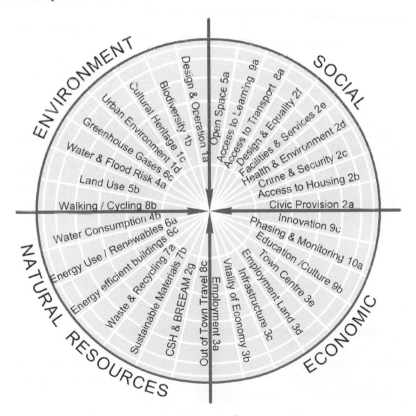

Figure 4.3   Northstowe sustainability performance diagram

Source: Arup (2007), reproduced courtesy of Gallagher Estates.

In order to promote wellbeing in the development of healthy and contented communities there are five fundamental steps to be taken in a continuing process:

Step 1 Set out the vision for a healthy and well-being community;
Step 2 Adopt a methodology for assessing and measuring the outcome;
Step 3 Undertake collaborative initiatives to deliver the vision;
Step 4 Consider periodically the effectiveness of the outcome; and
Step 5 Review and update the process.

For steps 1 and 2, the preparation of a 'Charter for Wellbeing', together with the preparation of quality of life indicators (QLIs) (approved and adopted by the promoters of a scheme, the local authorities, health providers and other public bodies and community representatives), can be the focus for the development of an expanded or new community. The use of QLIs and the scope for measuring and reporting on outcomes based on an analysis of various indices can be coupled with a user friendly approach such as the 'smiley faces' technique. The Charter would set out the key planning principles for the development of a healthy community and the QLIs. This would provide a technique for evaluating all progressive stages of a scheme against agreed wellbeing criteria including, for example, the promotion of walking and cycling to reduce car use and carbon emissions, building energy efficient homes, providing parks and open spaces, and enhancing employment opportunities to reduce inequalities (RTPI, 2009: 5).

For step 3, no amount of vision statements and policies and principles will deliver health and wellbeing without specific actions and initiatives being carried out, and effective and inclusive participation, representation, leadership and involvement within the community.

An important example from Scotland is the promotion of Healthy Living Centres to work alongside communities to influence services and develop programmes, which have made significant inroads to improve their health and wellbeing (Community Health Exchange, 2009). This initiative demonstrates that one of the most effective ways of addressing health inequalities and increasing the health and wellbeing of a community is to listen and act on needs identified by the communities themselves. Planning for physically active lifestyles to improve the quality of life and health – through increased walking and cycling activity, for example – forms an important part of local initiatives to be taken.

For steps 4 and 5, regular three- to five-year inclusive reviews, by representatives of all participants, of the progress made and the outcomes achieved will enable the effectiveness and value of the approach to be assessed for future action.

Wellbeing in new and expanded communities

The influence that urban planners have on social, physical and economic environments and the functioning of urban areas at a time of growth has been well documented (Barton and Tsouros, 2000).

The promotion and delivery of an adequate quantity of homes and a satisfactory level of wellbeing for new and expanded communities in an era of climate change was addressed by the growth areas policy of the former Labour government for a long-term programme of action to deliver sustainable communities and regeneration in both urban and rural areas (Office of the Deputy Prime Minister, 2003). The Coalition government's radical changes to these policies and the planning system were first announced in 2010, in an era of financial restraint with structural reform including abolition of regional housing targets and the introduction of local incentives for local authorities to encourage house-building (DCLG, 2010c).

Part of the former Labour government's response to major new communities was the proposal for 'Eco towns' to be exemplar developments of up to 20,000 homes designed to meet the highest standards of sustainability, including low and zero carbon technologies and good public transport (DCLG, 2007). In 2009, approval was given for the first wave of eco-town sites and 10,000 eco-homes were to be built in these four areas by 2016 (Directgov, 2009). The new homes and neighbourhoods were to be designed, planned and built to world-leading environmental standards. Funding was announced in March 2010 for potential second wave locations (DCLG, 2010a).

The concept of eco-towns was not without opposition, particularly where the plans encroached on green belt land, where they were seen as being unsustainable and likely to have an adverse affect on the regeneration of and provision of houses and employment in existing towns and cities. In July 2010, the Coalition government informed Local Authority leaders that the funding awards payable for eco-town projects in 2010/11 were to be reduced by 50 per cent. It made clear that the priority was to see that plans are well-supported locally and will achieve genuine improvements in sustainability. The government did not intend to designate or impose a solution on a particular area, and said it would not support an eco-town 'if the local community are opposed to it' (Regeneration and Renewal).

The intention for eco-towns that do proceed is to introduce the latest technology, including smart meters to track energy use, electric car charging points, properly insulated homes built to the highest standards, and systems for saving water and recycling and composting waste. Additional funding is to be made available to improve existing transport links, including dedicated routes for buses with real time travel information, green transport hubs and facilities for electric cars and bikes. New renewable energy projects will enable residents to take their green energy from natural sources. But what are the other ingredients of a future healthy, sustainable new community likely to be? In a recent report inspired by the former Labour government's eco-towns challenge panel, it was predicated for the attainment of eco-town status that they need to be based on exemplary place-making, master planning and architecture as the overarching principles that affect and define the settlement and its form. This will involve working with the landscape and the resources particular to the site, the design of healthy neighbourhoods, and a network of safe and attractive places, capable of supporting a variety of activities, enabling all residents to be physically active as a routine part of their daily life (BioRegional Development Group and CABE, 2008: 22).

These principles have been adopted for the proposed new town at Northstowe in Cambridgeshire, which is located five miles to the north west

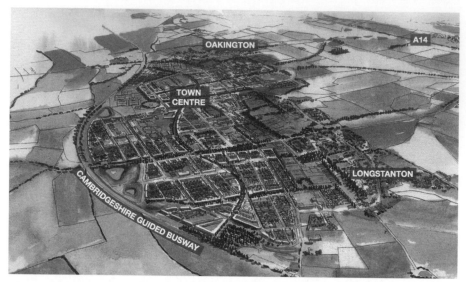

Figure 4.4   Proposed Northstowe New Town, Cambridgeshire

Reproduced courtesy of Gallagher Estates.

of Cambridge, off the A14. Exemplar master planning principles have been adopted for a sustainable new settlement for up to 10,000 dwellings, employment, a town centre, sports hubs and community facilities, six primary schools and a secondary school with over one third of the development area comprising public open space for formal and informal recreation (Figure 4.4).

Effective action on wellbeing and the physical environment involves the work of several professional groups, local authority officers and councillors – who all make a contribution to the shaping of the built and social environment, and have a key role to play in creating the favourable conditions for existing and new communities that will make them conducive to health, wellbeing and a high quality of life. The creation of neighbourhoods within these communities that promote and provide opportunities for active lifestyles would achieve enhanced wellbeing and a healthier outcome.

There is scope for better collaborative working. The RTPI recognized the importance of delivering healthy communities in the publication of a Good Practice Note in 2009, which sets out the context, the case for joint working between planning and health and planning principles for healthy communities (RTPI, 2009). The NHS London Health Urban Development Unit (HUDU) has been established as a specialist unit with a remit across London to promote better engagement at all levels between the health planning sectors. The HUDU provides advice to Primary Care Trusts (PCTs) and borough planners when new planning documents, policies or major developments are prepared in their area, basing this advice on a health and urban planning toolkit (NHS: HUDC, 2010). This approach may be capable of being more widely used.

Conclusion

It can be seen that, in order to increase standards of wellbeing and to improve the appearance, environmental standards and quality of our urban and rural areas, spatial planning in the twenty-first century has to be better connected to public health, and integrated and coordinated with the delivery of other local authority services.. Enhanced partnership and joint working between the professions would provide positive outcomes for health and wellbeing. The enthusiastic adoption of wellbeing as an objective by local authorities can be the universal ultimate objective and focus of all planning policy, and of the delivery of local services for new communities. It should be subject to a readily understood assessment as the primary analysis tool for policy and implementation.

The development of sustainable new communities can be promoted through the preparation of Wellbeing Charters setting out all key planning principles to be followed, owned and signed up to by all participants. A new methodology involving QLIs for assessing objective wellbeing coupled with an easy to understand assessment of subjective wellbeing such as the use of 'smiley faces' would provide an incentive and encouragement for full participation by the inhabitants of new and existing communities.

It is not, however, just a question of stating objectives, and assessing and measuring outcomes; it is also a matter of taking the positive actions necessary to achieve the desired outcomes. Arguably, the most important contribution will be centred on community-based initiatives and actions within existing or new communities, such as through the establishment of Healthy Living Centres. More cross-departmental working within local authorities and other agencies, with the full involvement of the inhabitants of an area, would help to achieve more efficient ways of delivering better health and wellbeing outcomes for everyone.

To follow these initiatives at a time of public spending restraint over the next few years will be challenging. However, the renewed emphasis on public and community involvement in local decisions affecting all aspects of people's lives will provide the opportunity for the concept of wellbeing to be a main determinant in local authority decisions. The potential benefits and advantages to the quality of life through the promotion of wellbeing are capable of being readily understood and agreed by all those who will be affected.

Given Coalition government policies to promote localism and grassroots involvement in public affairs, can local government really afford not to embrace wellbeing as an inspiring ambition and a driving force for change?

Bibliography

Arup (2007) 'Northstowe Sustainability Assessment Report'. Gallagher Longstanton Ltd and English Partnerships at www.northstowe.uk.com.

Barton. H. and Tsouros, C. (2000) *Healthy Urban Planning*, WHO Regional Office for Europe. London: Spon Press.

BioRegional Development Group and CABE (Commission for Architecture and the Built Environment) (2008) *What Makes an Eco-Town?* London: BioRegional Development Group and CABE.

Bond, M. (2003) 'The Pursuit of Happiness', *New Scientist*, 179(24152415): 40–3, October,, available on the webpages of Scott Falhman, Research Professor of Computer Science at Carnegie Mellon University at www.cs.cmu.edu/~sef/sefSmiley.htm (accessed 1 July 2010).

CABE (2010) 'Health and Wellbeing'. Available at www.cabe.org.uk/health

Chadwick, Edwin (1842) *Report on the Sanitary Condition of the Labouring Population of Great Britain.* Edinburgh: Edinburgh University Press and HMSO.

Clayden, P. (2009) *The Councillor.* Crayford, Kent: Shaw & Sons.

Community Health Exchange (CHEX) (2009) 'Breaking Through. Healthy Living Centres: Removing Barriers to Wellbeing'. Glasgow: CHEX. Available at www.chex.org.uk.

Conservative Party (2010) 'Open Source Planning Policy', Green Paper no. 14. London: Conservative Party.

DCLG (Department for Communities and Local Government) (2006a) 'Code for Sustainable Homes: A Step-Change in Sustainable Home Building Practice'. Wetherby: DCLG Publications. Available at www.communities.gov.uk.

DCLG (Department for Communities and Local Government) (2006b) 'Transferable Lessons from the New Towns'. Wetherby: DCLG Publications.

DCLG (Department for Communities and Local Government) (2007a) 'Homes for the Future: More Affordable, More Sustainable', Cm7191. Wetherby: DCLG Publications.

DCLG (Department for Communities and Local Government) (2007b) 'Eco-Towns Prospectus'. Wetherby: DCLG Publications.

DCLG (Department for Communities and Local Government) (2009) 'Local Strategic Partnerships (LSPs)', available on www.communities.gov.uk (accessed 29 July 2009).

DCLG (Department for Communities and Local Government) (2010a) 'Eco-Towns: Development of the Eco-Towns Policy'. Available at www.communities.gov.uk (accessed 9 March 2010).

DCLG (Department for Communities and Local Government) (2010b) 'Pickles Stops Unitary Councils in Exeter, Norwich and Suffolk'. Available at www.communities.gov.uk (accessed 26 May 2010).

DCLG (Department for Communities and Local Government) (2010c) 'Revoking Regional Strategies', available at www.communities.gov.uk (accessed 6 July 2010).

DCLG (Department for Communities and Local Government) (2010d) 'Communities and Local Government Structural Reform Plan'. London: CLG Publications.

DCLG (Department for Communities and Local Government) (2010e) 'Citizenship Survey: 2009–10 (April 2009–March 2010), England'. London: DCLG.

Defra (Department for the Environment, Food and Rural Affairs) (no date) 'Sustainable Development', available at sd.defra.gov.uk.

Defra (Department for the Environment, Food and Rural Affairs) (2010) 'Air Pollution: Action in a Changing Climate'. London: Defra. Available at www.defra.gov.uk.

Department for Business Innovation and Skills (2010) 'England's Regional Development Agencies', available at www.bis.gov.uk (accessed 1 July 2010).

Department of Health (2010) 'Health Impact Assessment'. Available at www.dh.gov.uk (accessed 2 July 2010).

DETR (Department of the Environment, Transport and the Regions) (1998) 'Modern Local Government: In Touch with the People'. London: DETR.

DETR (2000) 'Preparing Community Strategies'. London: DETR.

Directgov (2009) 'Green Light Given on Eco-Town Sites'. Available at www.direct.gov.uk (accessed 16 July 2009).

Dolan, P., Peasgood, T., Dixon, A., Knight, M., Phillips, D., Tsuchiya, A. and White, M. (2006) 'Research on the Relationship between Well-Being and Sustainable Development'. London: Defra.

Dyfed Powys Health Authority (2002) 'Health and Wellbeing in Powys: County Report 2002'. Camarthen: Dyfed Powys Health Authority.

Engels, F. (1844) *The Condition of the Working Class in England in 1844*. Leipzig: Oxford University Press.

Ereaut, G. and Whiting, R. (2008) 'What Do We Mean by "Wellbeing"? And Why Might It Matter?', *Linguistic Landscapes*: Research Report DCSF-RW073.

Falhman, S. (no date) 'Smiley Lore', available on the webpages of Scott Falhman, Research Professor of Computer Science at Carnegie Mellon University at www.cs.cmu.edu/~sef/sefSmiley.htm (accessed 1 July 2010).

Hansard Society (2010) 'The 7th Annual Audit of Political Engagement'. London: Hansard Society, available at www.hansardsociety.org.uk.

Harvey, W. Alexander (1906) *The Model Village and its Cottages. Bournville*. London. BT Batsford.

Healing Landscapes (2010) Available at www.healinglandscapes.org.

Hole, James (1866) *Homes of the Working Classes with Suggestions for their Improvement*. London: Longman.

Howard, Ebenezer (1898) *To-Morrow: A Peaceful Path to Real Reform*. London: Swan Sonnenschein.

Howard, Ebenezer (1902) *Garden Cities of To-Morrow*. London: 1902. Reprinted, edited with a Preface by F.J. Osborn and an Introductory Essay by Lewis Mumford. London: Faber & Faber, 1946.

HM Government (2005a) 'Securing the Future'. London: HMSO.

HM Government (2005b) 'Queen's Speech – Decentralisation and Localism Bill', Number 10 website. Available at www.number10.gov.uk/queens-speech/2010/05 (accessed 25 May 2010).

HM Government (2009) 'Putting the Frontline First: Smarter Government'. London: HMSO.

HM Government (2010a) 'The Coalition: Our Programme for Government'. London: Cabinet Office.

HM Government (2010b) Cabinet Office website CAB 059-10. Available at www.cabinetoffice.gov.uk (accessed 18 May 2010).

HM Government (2010c) Citizenship Survey: 2009–10 (April 2009–March 2010), England.

HM Treasury (2010) 'Action to Tackle Poor Value for Money and Unfunded Spending Commitments', Press Notice PN13/10, 17 June. London: HM Treasury. Available at www.hm-treasury.gov.uk.

HM Treasury and CLG (Communities and Local Government) (2010) 'Total Place: A Whole Approach to Public Services'. London: HM Treasury.

HM Treasury and the Department for Business Innovation and Skills (2011) 'The Plan for Growth', March. London: HM Treasury.

HRH The Prince of Wales (1989) *A Vision of Britain*. London/New York: Doubleday. See www.duchyofcornwall.org/designanddevelopment_poundbury.htm.

Howard, Ebenezer (1898) *Tomorrow: A Peaceful Path to Real Reform*. Swan Sonnenschein.

Invest Milton Keynes (2007) 'From New Town to International City. How, Why, What, When, Where', available at www.investmiltonkeynes.com.

James, David (2004) 'Salt, Sir Titus, First Baronet (1803–1876)', *Oxford Dictionary of National Biography*. Oxford: Oxford University Press. See www.oxforddnb.com/view/article/24565.

Le Corbusier (Re-issued June 1987) *The City of Tomorrow and Its Planning*, trans. by Frederick Etchells. New York: Dover Publications.

Lloyd Wright, Frank (1932) *The Disappearing City*. New York: W.F. Payson.

Local Democracy, Economic Development and Construction Act (2009) London: HMSO.

Local Government Act (2000) London: HMSO.

Local Government Bill (2010) London: HMSO.

Local Government and Public Involvement in Health Act 2007 London: HMSO.

Localism Bill (2010) London: HMSO.

Meteorological Office (2009) 'Act on CO_2 Warming: Climate Change – The Facts'. Exeter: Meteorological Office.

National Assembly for Wales (2009) 'Inquiry into Local Government Scrutiny and Overview Arrangements', Health, Wellbeing and Local Government Committee, March 2009. Cardiff Bay: National Assembly for Wales. Available at www.assemblywales.org.

NHS: Health Scotland (2007) 'How Do Councillors Improve Health and Community Wellbeing?'. NHS: Health Scotland. Available at www.healthscotland.com.

NHS: HUDU (London Healthy Urban Development Unit) (2010) 'Healthier and More Sustainable Communities'. London: NHS, HUDU. Available at www.healthy urbandevelopment.nhs.uk.

Number 10 website (25 May 2010) Available at www.number10.gov.ukOffice of the Deputy Prime Minister (2003) 'Sustainable Communities: Building for the Future'. London: ODPM.

Office of the Deputy Prime Minister (2005) 'Sustainable Communities: People Places and Prosperity'. London: HMSO.

Planning and Compulsory Purchase Act (2004) London: HMSO.

Regeneration and Renewal (2010) 'Government Deals Blow to Warwickshire Eco-Town Plan', available at www.regen.net (accessed 1 July 2010).

Richardson, Benjamin Ward (1876) *Hygeia, A City of Health*. Basingstoke: Macmillan.

RTPI (Royal Town Planning Institute) (2009) 'Delivering Healthy Communities', RTPI Good Practice Note 5, June, available from http://www.rtpi.org.uk/.

Stewart, J. (2003) *Modernising British Local Government*. Basingstoke: Palgrave Macmillan.

Steuer, N. and Marks, N. (2007) *Local Wellbeing: Can We Measure It?* London: Young Foundation.

Tizard, J. (2010) 'Can Total Place Survive?', available at www.publicfinance.co.uk (accessed 1 June 2010).

Welsh Assembly Government (2007) 'Health, Social Care and Wellbeing Strategies Guidance'. Cardiff: Welsh Assembly Government. Available at www.wales.gov.uk.

Wellbeing and Children and Young People

Sarah Lloyd-Jones and Duncan Holtom

This chapter looks at why societies are particularly concerned about the well-being of children and young people. It also explores how protecting the well-being of children has come to be seen as important – both in its own right, as the action of a civilized society, and as an investment in the future. It considers what constitutes wellbeing for children and young people, and why children and young people's wellbeing has risen up the political agenda and captured the popular imagination. It examines the dichotomy between society's wish to protect the wellbeing of the vulnerable child and to protect its own wellbeing from the anti-social adolescent. We also examine the extent to which the state can enable wellbeing, and the 'responsibility' of state, family and children and young people themselves to promote wellbeing and protect against 'ill-being'.

A brief history of childhood

The very concept of childhood and youth or adolescence as a state distinct from adulthood is relatively modern. Phillipe Aries' influential work *Centuries of Childhood* (1962) argued that, in the medieval world, children and young people were simply 'little adults'. Poor life expectancy amongst the young and the struggle for survival experienced by most of the population meant that childhood was, in modern terms, very short. The sooner a child could become a net contributor to the household the better, and adults had little interest in preserving childhood beyond what was absolutely necessary. Aries contends that it was not until the thirteenth to sixteenth centuries that an increasing separation between the adult and child world emerged, as did concerns about the wellbeing, thinking and behaviour of 'children', and later of 'young people', as distinct groups. Since its 'invention', childhood has grown in importance and length so that, between the beginning of the nineteenth century and the current day, the length of childhood doubled to the point where, by 2010, many policies relating to children and young people look at 21 years, or even 25 years, as the transition age to adulthood.

The emergence of childhood as a distinct phase was accompanied by shifting and competing conceptions of children and young people either as potential victims, whose welfare – what we would now think of as wellbeing – needs protection from the evils of adult society; or, as potential threats to society because, until disciplined and socialized into 'responsible' adults, their immaturity means they threaten the welfare and wellbeing of others. Although societal attitudes have shifted between these two polarized positions, in many ways they represent two sides of the same coin. This is because many of the behaviours and experiences, such as drug and alcohol abuse, criminality and anti-social behaviour – which, as outlined in the third section, are now considered detrimental to children and young people's wellbeing – are also the behaviours that threaten others.

As explored in the following section, the competing ideas of innocence and deviance/threat – rooted in the notion of the child as both a vulnerable and an incomplete adult: immature, unsocialized and untrained, in need of care and control/discipline – shape modern concerns about children and young people's wellbeing. Concerns about teenage parenthood provide an excellent illustration of these tensions and the competing conceptions of childhood and youth in the twenty-first century. A wide range of political and social perspectives characterize teenage parents as:

- irresponsible parasites expecting an over-indulgent state to provide the support they need to bring up their child (see Murray, 1990; Williamson, 1997, for discourses on an 'underclass'); or
- incomplete adults, unable to provide the nurture and security needed for a child's wellbeing, leading to a need to 'protect' the child from their inadequate parenting (for discourses on inadequate parenting, see Desforge and Abouchaar, 2003; Katz *et al.*, 2007); or
- young mothers whose own wellbeing and prematurely interrupted youth compromise them by their attendant impacts (for discourses on social exclusion and feminism, see Tabberer *et al.*, 2000).

(See Duncan *et al.*, 2010, for a full discussion of these issues.)

These competing positions illustrate some of the tensions between the wellbeing of the individual and that of the state (or society). For some, supporting the young mother in bringing up her child is necessary to protect both her wellbeing and that of her child (Tabberer *et al.*, 2000) However, for others, the introduction of support encourages these behaviours, increasing the numbers of teenage parents and vulnerable children, exposing others to harm and increasing the costs to the state (Murray, 1990).

The increasing role of the state as protector and promoter of wellbeing

Until the nineteenth century, the state did little to intervene in children's wellbeing, seeing it as exclusively the responsibility of the child's parent or guardian to ensure its health and happiness. In 1802, the first Factory Act started a pattern that would develop over the next two hundred years of increasing state legislation to protect children and young people from the adults who controlled their lives, and to protect their wellbeing. That Act set out to regulate the employment of children but, as well as forbidding the employment of those under 9 years old and restricting the hours children could work, it also placed a duty on employers to provide children with access to education, protection from disease and spiritual guidance. Over the subsequent decades, increasingly interventionist legislation moved from guidance to enforcement. By 1880, all children aged between 5 and 10 years were required to attend school (Elementary Education Act, 1880), whether their parents wanted them to or not, and by 1944 schooling was compulsory until 15 years of age (1944 Education Act). The nineteenth century also saw the state taking other steps to protect children from their parents. In 1889, for example, the 'children's charter' was adopted, the first law allowing police to intervene between parent and child to stop cruelty. Four years later, it became illegal to deny a sick child medical attention and, in 1908, the Punishment of Incest Act made sexual abuse within families illegal.

In the twentieth century, changes in public opinion became increasingly powerful drivers of the state's response. Legalization, literature and cultural attitudes alternated between concern to protect children (and young people) from society and concerns to protect society from children and young people, by disciplining and controlling them. State intervention in children and young people's wellbeing moved from being led by the type of reformers who pushed for the first Factory Acts to more general public attitudinal changes to the state's responsibilities concerning children. Public concerns about youth as a threat, for example, have made it politically easier to focus upon 'corrective' responses, looking at ways of 'controlling' young people and their anti-social or risky behaviour. Aries describes the modern world as 'obsessed by the physical, moral and sexual problems of childhood' (1962: 411). In contrast, public responses to cruelty have also become major policy drivers around children and young people, with key cases leading to new legislation. Dennis O'Neill's death at the hands of his foster carers in 1945 led to the first Children Act in 1948, which required local authorities in the UK to have structures in place specifically for the protection of children. The death of Victoria Climbié led, in England, to the Green Paper 'Every Child Matters', and the 2004 Children Act, which introduced new duties to safeguard, protect and promote children's well-being. More broadly, since the 1960s the 'deficit' model of childhood has been increasingly challenged, and children and young people have become increasingly defined as individuals with rights, rather than being defined by the adult attributes they lacked (Heywood, 2001).

In the second half of the twentieth century, the children's rights agenda became increasingly important. This agenda represents a response to both the 'child as victim' and 'youth as deviant' policy drivers by aiming to regulate the state's 'paternalistic' approach to caring for the vulnerable by setting out a series of rights and, by so doing, also to curb its powers to punish. The rights agenda also leads much of the policy work around children and sustainable development – seeing sustainable development in the context of young people's inheritance and, where possible, seeking to capture their interests and embed habits and behaviour that raise awareness of, and promote, sustainability. For example, Eco-Schools is an international programme run by the Foundation for Environmental Development that seeks to involve children and young people in assessing the environmental performance of their school.

These national changes have been mirrored by international changes. Landmarks include the League of Nations adoption of the Geneva Declaration of the Rights of the Child in 1924, the United Nations General Assembly's adoption of the Universal Declaration of Human Rights in 1948, and the United Nations Convention on the Rights of the Child (UNCRC) in 1989. As a consequence, the twentieth century was dubbed by some the 'century of the child' (after Kay, 1900).

Inequality, development and well-being

As societies have learned more about the complexities of human psychology, physical development and behaviour, they have sought to 'correct' social and health problems in adult society through managing the development of the child. This represents a richer, more complex (Foucauldian) notion of 'discipline' and 'control' that goes beyond the earlier notion of imposing adult rules and behaviour on 'immature' children to shaping the very development of the person. Increasingly, the state's identification of the essential elements of a 'good' childhood, make the state interest in the wellbeing of the child uniquely defined. It could be argued that the Jesuit motto 'Give me the child until he is seven years and I will show you the man' (attributed to St Francis Xavier) underpins much of modern day thinking and policy about young people and children.

These changes in our understanding of the impact of childhood upon human development – together with the gradual erosion in confidence in the effectiveness of the family, or at least some families, to adequately shape and 'socialize' children and young people – mean that, in the twenty-first century, the impact of childhood upon lifelong wellbeing has become a major driver for policy development and intervention in the life of the child. During the second half of the twentieth century, the social structures that historically helped families to 'socialize' children lost their scope, or will, to tell people how to live their lives – a gap the state has increasingly sought to fill. As the state's concern about the capacity of some families to raise healthy well-adjusted citizens has risen, this, in turn, has led to the evolution of new and increasing roles for institutions such as the school, health and social welfare services, and the juvenile justice system, giving them responsibility to supplement or even replace parental roles in helping train and discipline children (Bessant and Watts, 2007).

The concern over the effectiveness of families has been sharpened by social, economic and cultural changes. The power of religion, society and class to establish and monitor social 'norms' was gradually displaced over the second half of the twentieth century as society moved towards a notion of 'individualism' (Furlong and Cartmel, 1997; Catan, 2004). In this new 'risk society' (Beck, 1992), children and young people were increasingly required to become active agents, architects of their own futures, actively navigating risks and exploiting opportunities, This increased demand upon individual agency (Giddens, 1991) has raised the emphasis placed upon the role of childhood as a preparation for the challenges of adult life and has increased the impact of the choices made by children and young people in childhood upon their adult lives.

In theory, young people who used to be bound by class, locality and education to follow their parents' lives now have much greater freedom to choose their own journey through life. Even the 16-year-old school leaver with no qualifications – and therefore the least amount of choice – is now faced with a series of options (Green *et al.*, 2001) and this has been a rapid change. In 1988, more than half of school leavers went straight into a job (Furlong and Cartmel, 1997) but, by the end of the 1990s, school leavers were able to select from options such as training, further education and work experience programmes, from which a job was by no means the most likely outcome.

But these benefits are unequally distributed and come at a price. Economic, social and political changes have created new opportunities for young people, but have also exposed them to much greater risks (Beck, 1992) – and the capacity to exploit the new opportunities whilst managing these increased risks is unequally distributed. Researchers such as Antony Giddens have described how human agency shapes our capacity both to create and to use new structures (Giddens, 1991). To function in a 'risk society', young people have to become decisionmakers, planners and strategists, and be able to exploit services and capitalize on resources. Policies increasingly require the young person to be an active participant, a decisionmaker who is able to plan for the future and map their own needs. In order to prosper in such a society, young people need to be 'reflexive', better able to exploit opportunities and manage risks (Giddens, 1991: Beck, 1992; Margo and Dixon, 2006). It is clear that some young people are better equipped and supported to do this than others. Young people's capacity to exploit opportunities and avoid the risks created by economic, social and political change depends upon how they approach those opportunities and risks (their orientation to them), and the resources they can access.

Concerns about inequality – and, in particular, inequality of opportunity – have also been major drivers of state policy. For example, since the introduction of compulsory schooling, and particularly since the 1960s, state education has come to be seen as the key structural tool for tackling socio-economic disadvantage and for promoting social equality (Hodgson, 1999). Even more broadly, schools are seen as the place to develop good citizenship, promote healthy lifestyles and concern for the environment. They are a preparation for adulthood, and Herford (1957), Kohlberg and Gilligan (1971) and Piaget (1972) all describe early school leaving as a problem for society because it curtails opportunities for systematic learning involving cognitive and moral development. The 1944 Education Act set out to change the fact that children from working class homes consistently achieved least from education and, subsequently, took the poorest paid employment (Carter, 1966). Compulsory education has been in a process of almost continual change ever since, with all of the major changes being focused as much on social equality as on education.

Well-becoming: the legacy of child wellbeing for adult life

The increasing interest in wellbeing over the life course is encapsulated in concepts such as 'well-becoming'. In modern society, childhood wellbeing is seen both as an issue for the child and for the adult that child will become. The legacy of childhood wellbeing for adult life is both structural and functional. As we explored in earlier sections, childhood has, for most people, a direct impact on the employment they will have and the life they will live, linking discourses about child and adolescent wellbeing to those of the child poverty and equalities agendas. It also impacts on how happy people will be with that life and their capacity to cope with adversity, linking these same discourses to the happiness, resilience and mental health agendas.

Socio-economic disadvantage can have a negative impact on education and the evidence is that leaving school with poor qualifications is a strong indicator of poverty in adult life (Feinstein et al., 2007) which is, as we have seen, a significant factor for wellbeing. Bivand's 2003 report on the Youth Cohort Studies shows, for example, that the likelihood of an 18-year-old not being in education, training or work is much higher if they have truanted in year 11; were excluded from school in year 10 or 11and/or have no qualification higher than level 2 . Most people with no qualifications at the age of 19 will not have acquired any by the age of 25, and those aged 25–50 with no qualifications face a markedly higher risk of unemployment, economic inactivity and life on low pay (Kenway et al., 2005; cf. Macdonald and Marsh, 2005), all contra-indications for wellbeing. Ill-being in childhood, especially around social and emotional development (HM Treasury, 2007) is now seen as a key predictor of problems in adulthood, with some studies suggesting they may be even more powerful predictors of outcomes than literacy and numeracy (Margo and Dixon, 2006; Feinstein et al., 2007).

As has been explored, some young people fail to thrive in education, and research is increasingly focusing on the importance of resilience in enabling individuals to cope with life. This research sees resilience as both a function (i.e. wellbeing provides resilience) and a protector (i.e. resilience provides wellbeing) of wellbeing, and marks the importance of childhood as the time when individuals develop resilience. The Resilience Research Centre (RRC) describes resilience as the capacity of individuals to find the psychological, social, cultural and physical resources to sustain their wellbeing while facing significant difficulties, and the capacity, individually and collectively, to negotiate the provision of these resources in a meaningful way (Resilience Project (no date)).

In some ways, the focus upon resilience mirrors debates over the status of the child as victim or sinner. It places greater emphasis upon individual agency and resources, and less upon the role of the family and state in the exercising of resilience; that is, how young people behave and the choices they make. However, such focus also recognizes the importance of the family and state in promoting the capacity of the individual to behave and make choices that protect wellbeing. For example, not all young people with poor resilience will fail to achieve qualifications. If there are others around them, such as parents, who are 'managing' their experiences effectively, they may emerge from childhood with good qualifications but still with little personal resilience.

Redefining the role of the state and family

As outlined in the previous sections, the state has adopted an increasingly interventionist role in childhood in the last two hundred years (Batty, 2009). The state has sought, initially, to protect children and young people from exploitation, and has gradually included elements of 'the good' childhood, such as those prescribed by the United Nations Convention on the Rights of the Child (UNCRC) (1989). Policy towards children and young people's wellbeing is therefore distinctive: in part, because of the level of state investment and the responsibility the state takes upon itself for their wellbeing. Nevertheless, evidence of trends in wellbeing, which we discuss further in the following section, suggests a mixed picture and, as we outline in this section, the state has therefore developed and redefined its role.

By the end of the first decade of the twenty-first century, there has been a decided policy shift away from the state seeking directly to protect and meet the needs of the child towards supporting the family as the primary tool for promoting child wellbeing (Bacon *et al.*, 2010). This has been driven, in part, by the evidence that the large amount of public spending on children and young people is failing to produce results in many areas of child wellbeing. For example, an Organisation for Economic Co-operation and Development report, 'Doing Better for Children' (OECD, 2009), compared public spending and policies on children with key indicators of wellbeing, (including education, health, housing, family incomes and quality of school life) in all OECD countries. The report found that, on average, governments spend US$125,000 on children but that spending, of itself, is an insufficient guarantee of ensuring child wellbeing. The United States, for example, spends more than the OECD average on children, and yet US children do worse in areas such as health, with infant mortality the 4th highest, child mortality the 5th highest, and education the 7th lowest across all 34 OECD countries. The report concluded that, if they wished to reduce social inequalities and improve child wellbeing, governments need to invest more in the first six years of children's lives, which currently attract only one quarter of total public spending (and much less in the US). The UK is described as spending more on early years than the average for OECD countries, but less than it spends on children aged over six years, mainly because of the cost of compulsory education. The report suggests a need to move away from a generic spend on children, which sees the majority of government money going on compulsory education, to more targeted interventions at an earlier age incorporating family support.

There is an increasing recognition that there are limits to what the state can achieve in ensuring wellbeing for children and young people. Rather than intervening directly, providing support to build a family's capacity and resilience is increasingly being seen to be the most effective way of promoting child wellbeing. This approach includes recognition that the wellbeing of the adults caring for a child has a direct and potentially lasting impact on the child, and that tackling one without dealing with the other is likely to be ineffective. This focus on the family as the source of wellbeing is seen as reversing a trend towards state management of childhood.

Defining and measuring wellbeing for children and young people

The state's role in defining and promoting the concept of a 'good' childhood has increasingly become linked to a holistic view of a child's wellbeing. As the state has assumed progressively more responsibility for the wellbeing of children, the first decade of the twenty-first century has seen an increasing interest in the development of measures and tools to try to assess how well it is doing (e.g. Land *et al.*, 2006; UNICEF, 2007; Welsh Assembly Government, 2008; CPAG, 2009; Children's Society, no date).

As described in Chapter 2, wellbeing can be defined both as a state and as an experience; that is, subjective wellbeing (reflected in questions about one's satisfaction with life) and a set of conditions (the factors, such as good health, that enable a person to experience wellbeing). These two conceptions are reflected in a series of studies into children and young people's wellbeing, including those undertaken by UNICEF, the Welsh Assembly Government, York University and the Children's Society.

The UNICEF report, 'Child Poverty in Perspective: An Overview of Child Well-Being' (2007), draws upon data on 21 industrialized countries. Wellbeing is defined in relation to six dimensions:

- material well-being;
- health and safety;
- educational well-being;
- family and peer relationships;
- behaviours and risks; and
- subjective well-being.

The average rank position of all six measures is used to give an overall ranking. Each domain is treated as of equal importance, as are the individual indicators for each of the six dimensions. They find that 'No single dimension of well-being stands as a reliable proxy for child well-being as a whole and several OECD countries find themselves with widely differing rankings for different dimensions of child well-being' (UNICEF, 2007: 5). Wellbeing is defined as a relative concept. In total, it draws upon 40 distinct indicators described as 'relevant to children's lives and children's rights'. The definition is rooted in the availability of data, and the report asserts that 'the definition of child well-being that permeates the report is one that will also correspond to the views and the experience of a wide public' (UNICEF, 2007: 5). The report argues that the reason for measuring wellbeing is to inform policy responses to improve it, by aiding monitoring of progress, raising the profile of wellbeing, enabling accountability, helping inform resource allocations and showing what is achievable.

The Welsh Assembly Government's 'Children and Young People's Well-Being Monitor' (2008) also uses a multidimensional conception of wellbeing focused upon seven dimensions that broadly mirror those in the UN Convention on the Rights of the Child:

- *Dimension 1*: The Early Years – having 'a flying start in life';
- *Dimension 2*: Access to Education, Training and Learning Opportunities – a comprehensive range of education and learning opportunities;
- *Dimension 3*: Health, Freedom from Abuse and Exploitation – the best possible health and freedom from abuse, victimization and exploitation;
- *Dimension 4*: Access to Play, Leisure, Sport and Culture – access to play, leisure, sporting and cultural activities;
- *Dimension 5*: Children are Listened to, Treated with Respect and have their Race and Cultural Identity recognized – being listened to, treated with respect, and having their race and cultural identity recognized;
- *Dimension 6*: Safe Home and Community – a safe home, and a community that supports physical and emotional wellbeing; and
- *Dimension 7*: Child Poverty – not disadvantaged by poverty.

As in the UNICEF report, these dimensions are informed by the UNCRC and, by enabling monitoring of wellbeing, the report aims to raise awareness, and inform and measure the impact of policy. It offers a relative measure; relative to earlier periods and, in some cases, other UK nations.

The York University study, *Wellbeing of Children in the UK*, (Bradshaw *et al.*, 2006) commissioned by Save the Children, also uses a multidimensional approach, based upon 61 indicators. It reports results for each indicator, and also groups indicators under 10 themes:

- poverty;
- demography;
- physical health;
- lifestyle;
- mental health;
- education;

- housing and neighbourhood;
- time and space;
- substitute care; and
- crime.

A key message is summarized for each indicator. It also adopts a relative measure, comparing earlier periods and, in some cases, the UK nations and other European nations and the genders.

In 2006, the Children's Society commissioned the *Good Childhood Inquiry* (Layard and Dunn, 2009), which set out to gather the perspectives of children and young people themselves on what constitutes wellbeing. Over a period of two years, the Inquiry gathered evidence from over 10,000 children and young people (opinions, thoughts, pictures and suggestions), together with contributions from adults, to define what makes a good childhood. The Inquiry report grouped the findings under seven themes:

- family;
- friends;
- lifestyle;
- values;
- schooling;
- mental health; and
- inequalities.

The Children's Society went on to produce the report 'Understanding Children's Well-Being' (Rees *et al.*, 2010) and launched a programme to measure wellbeing against the indicators identified.

Current public attitudes

All the studies cited above illustrate the increasing interest in children and young people's wellbeing, and also provide evidence that, on many measures, their wellbeing is not good and that there are persistent inequalities. This, in turn, is seen as both a symptom and a cause of a wider social malaise. The proposition that Britain is 'broken' resonates with the public (*Economist*, 2010; see also Margo and Dixon, 2006). It encompasses the duality of thinking about children and young people explored in this chapter: concerns about children and young people as a threat, and concerns about young people as victims. Concerns about children and young people as a threat are reflected in a focus on youth crime, antisocial behaviour and teenage pregnancy, and underpin notions of so called 'feral' youth and the 'youth underclass'. Concerns about young people as victims are reflected in a focus on educational disengagement and underachievement, unemployment, mental ill health and family breakdown, and underpin discourses about the 'lost generation' and the numbers of young people who are not in education, employment or training. Many of these aspects – such as drug and alcohol misuse, including 'binge drinking' – transcend the duality and reflect concerns over youth as both a threat and victim – or as both symptom and cause of a 'broken' society.

The evidence

A news article summed up the dilemma as follows, 'Given less crime, less killing, fewer teenage mums, far fewer fags, perhaps a bit less drink and drugs: why is it that the idea of "broken Britain" rings true with so many, when it seems far from reality?' (*Economist*, 2010). It is suggested that there are various reasons for the gap between statistics and popular feeling: suspicion of official statistics (people do not believe that rates are actually falling); faster progress in other countries (the importance of comparative wellbeing); or a shift from local to national newspapers, so people are exposed to stories from throughout the UK, at which scale bad things are always likely to be happening. An example of the gap between perception and reality can be seen with teenage pregnancy, a popular barometer or measure of the 'state' of youth. Rates of teenage pregnancy have steadily declined since 1967 (when abortions were legalized) and a young woman aged between 15 and 19 today is about half as likely to have a baby in her teens as her grandmother was. This does not resonate with the popular imagination though: approximately one in 300 teenagers is a teenage parent, yet opinion polls suggest the public believe four out of ten teenagers have children (*Economist*, 2010).

Overall, the evidence on trends in children and young people's wellbeing is equivocal. On some measures, children and young people's wellbeing has declined in relative terms, compared with earlier periods; yet, on others it has improved. For example, in 2005, the UK government-funded Nuffield Foundation study *Time Trends in Adolescent Mental Health* found a dramatic rise across a series of measures relating to anxiety, depression and conduct problems among 11–15 year-olds between 1974 and 1999. In children, young people and adults, good mental health is increasingly seen as a necessary condition for wellbeing. An update to the study to 2004 (Hagell, 2010) found that problems were levelling off and, of nine different measures of mental health, eight had improved since 1999 or stayed the same.

Generalizations hide increasing polarization in which, while aspects of wellbeing may be improving overall, it is improving faster for some groups than others; in some cases, trends diverge. So, for example, overall alcohol consumption is rising and young drinkers are drinking greater quantities than ever, but the number of young people who abstain completely from alcohol is also rising (*Economist*, 2010). Similarly, some young people are accessing a more open and diverse labour market than they ever have. However, the positive changes in employment opportunities that create this diversity at a national and European level (Gangl, 2002) mask an increase in disadvantage at a local level, whereby young people with no or low qualifications have fewer employment chances than ever. This polarization can have a significant impact on overall wellbeing, since people rate their happiness and satisfaction with life relative to others around them.

As we have seen, individualism has led to a loss of common experience amongst groups within society, leading to an increased requirement for personal resilience, self-efficacy (see Beck, 1992, and Schoon, 2006, on the risk society) and emotional and social intelligence (Goleman, 1995). Even for those young people with higher-level qualifications, there is less certainty than there used to be as increasing attainment and participation in further and higher education means that the premiums secured by high-level qualifications at a UK level are not as significant as they used to be (Furlong and Cartmel, 2005; Leitch, 2007). As a result of this, a minority of young people will find themselves living back at home with parents and unemployed after completing degrees (Schneider, 2000).

Factors that influence wellbeing

Both general and specific factors driving the trends in wellbeing have been discussed in the previous section. The general factors affect a range of indicators, while the specific ones affect only one or a handful of them. The selection of which indicators to include and which to exclude in measures of wellbeing, therefore, influences the salience of particular policies or causes in shaping children and young people's wellbeing. For example, different measures of children and young people's health can be used, ranging from teenage pregnancy rates to rates of immunization amongst young children. The factors affecting these measures of wellbeing are very different.

Some indicators of wellbeing, such as rates of immunization amongst young children, relate to the circumstances in which a child or young person find themselves and the choices others, predominately adults and the state, make on their behalf. Other elements, such as engaging in risky behaviour, are ostensibly within their control, but there remains a lively debate over the extent to which children and young people exercise agency and freely make these choices, and the extent to which they are externally determined (see structure versus agency in Rudd and Evans, 1998 and post-structuralist accounts in Lloyd-Jones, 2005).

A number of general or underlying causes that influence the different dimensions of wellbeing have been identified: genetics, increasing inequality, poverty, social change, capability and resilience, and temperament.

Genetics: Many important aspects of wellbeing – such as aspects of health and disposition – are, in part, determined by genetics. So, for example, educational attainment may depend partly upon IQ, which is itself partly heritable. This does not mean there is a simple causal relationship, and it is often the interplay between genes and the environment ('genes × environment') that determines outcomes (Rutter *et al.*, 2006).

Increasing inequality: The Institute of Fiscal Studies has shown that household income rose by an average of 2 per cent per year between 1996–97 and 2007–08, but on most measures it ended up more unequally distributed than at any time since at least 1961. There is strong evidence that comparative health and wealth has as strong an impact on wellbeing as other objective measures. In 1974, Richard Easterlin famously demonstrated that, above a certain level, rising income does not increase happiness (the Easterlin Paradox), suggesting that wealth, by itself, is not a sufficient measure of wellbeing. More recently, in the influential work *The Spirit Level*, Wilkinson and Pickett (2009) argued that increasing inequality leads to status competition and increased anxiety (with negative consequences upon wellbeing).

Poverty: Although wealth has been shown not to be a sufficient measure of wellbeing, there is a strong relationship between wellbeing and child poverty. Measures of wellbeing often include child poverty as a component, so there is an element of circularity here, but even if the dimension is stripped out as an independent measure, child poverty is strongly associated with lower levels of wellbeing (although not seen as an adequate proxy of wellbeing (UNICEF, 2007)). Causes of child poverty are complex and linked to the poverty of families which is, in turn, linked to rates of employment, pay and the benefits structure. Again, there are issues of equality, in that children born into poor families are significantly more likely than others to be poor as adults (Margo and Dixon, 2006).

Social change: A key factor in wellbeing is the quality of social interaction experienced. Technological advances and improvements in housing provision have contributed to a life increasingly spent indoors and to an increase in virtual interaction, through mobile phones and the internet. Television and computer games can also contribute to isolation and a limiting of collective or group experiences (Putnam, 2000). As already highlighted, there has been a shift from community or collective experiences to the individualization of the risk society (Beck, 1992). Whilst this has created greater choice and freedom for some, those choices are inevitably constrained by the range of options available to each individual (Giddens, 1999) and their capacity to use them effectively.

Capability and resilience: Children and young people's thinking and behaviour have an impact upon their wellbeing. Their capabilities (including their cognitive, social and emotional skills, and consequently their resilience – that is their ability to cope with adversity) vary considerably (Feinstein *et al.*, 2007).

Temperament: This also has a significant impact upon the subjective dimension of wellbeing. For example, some people are happier and more optimistic than others, even when their conditions of life are the same. This, in turn, may also influence their thinking and behaviour, and the consequent conditions of their life.

In addition to these general or meta causes, there is a range of specific factors linked to individual indicators of wellbeing. For example, immunization rates have been influenced by media coverage of scares over vaccines such as MMR; but this had no impact on other dimensions of wellbeing.

Conclusion

This chapter has shown how, as conceptions of childhood and adolescence emerged, so did concerns about the wellbeing of children and young people.

These concerns have been rooted both in the deficit concept of youth (in which young people are seen as incomplete or 'lesser' in terms of maturity and social-ization) and in an idealized conception of childhood (as an age of innocence before the 'fall' of adulthood), with children seen as good, but vulnerable, and therefore in need of protection. These conceptions of childhood as a time of both vulnerability and deficit have raised the profile and importance of chil-dren's wellbeing. There is now increasing consensus on the multi-dimensional conception of wellbeing (although there is still continuing debate over the precise measures or indicators), and wellbeing discourses have become focused upon five core issues:

- concerns over a child's or young person's quality of life now (wellbeing in the present);
- the impact of a child's or young person's choices, behaviour and quality of life on their future as an adult (wellbeing in the future, sometimes described as well-becoming);
- the complexity of wellbeing, as reflected in differences in the wellbeing of different groups and in trends in each dimension of wellbeing;
- the wellbeing of children and young people as an indicator of the quality and 'health' of a society; and
- the role of the individual, family and state in influencing wellbeing in both the present and the future.

The nature of these issues illustrates why the role of the state in children and young people's wellbeing has developed so radically over the twentieth and into the twenty-first centuries. Children and young people's wellbeing has come increasingly to be seen as a public issue and one that the state must address. Alternatively, it is being seen as an investment strategy for future social wellbeing (with the idea that happy well-adjusted children turn into happy, well-adjusted adults); as a protective strategy for current social wellbe-ing (one that seeks to mitigate the wider impacts of ill-being seen in delin-quency and other problems); and as a proxy-indicator of civilization, (showing that the state is capable of protecting the vulnerable and the weak).

The picture that emerges of children and young people's wellbeing is complex. All too frequently, measures of wellbeing are showing that the state has succeeded in promoting some aspects of wellbeing, but has failed to promote or protect other aspects. There are also marked differences in the wellbeing of different groups of children and young people, especially seen in relation to child poverty and socio-economic inequalities. For example: many of the objective measures of wellbeing, such as physical health, are improving; children and young people have more legal protection than ever before; chil-dren are more likely to survive childhood and emerge as healthy and educated; and children now have their right to be listened to and treated with respect enshrined in an internationally adopted charter (UNCRC, 1989). There is also a widespread recognition of the importance of the early years of a child's life for cognitive, social and emotional development. However, other measures of wellbeing, such as mental health, appear to be declining; and fears about the wellbeing of children and young people are probably higher than they have ever been. For many, this constitutes a failure of the state, society and the family.

The concerns about childhood wellbeing, initially rooted in a perceived need to protect children, have grown as our understanding of the formative importance of the early years of a person's life has also grown. Studies of social inequalities show that a child's family circumstances still presents the best predictor of the kind of adult life they will lead. Such studies also show that a child born to affluent, well-educated parents is more likely to become an affluent and well-educated adult than a child born in poverty to poorly-educated parents. These formative experiences are seen as crucial to the development of resilience and, therefore, to a large degree, the potential to experience wellbeing throughout their lifetime. This, along with a need to protect the vulnerable from exploitation, means that societies have increasingly seen child wellbeing as a matter for state intervention. However, this chapter has also shown how investment in public services has had a limited impact on ensuring wellbeing, failing to break the patterns of inherited disadvantage that lead to the intergenerational transmission of both wellbeing and ill-being. This failure has led to societies looking in greater depth at the root causes of well-being and ill-being – including why, for example, poverty leads to children being less successful in the school system. The importance of wellbeing, both as a pre-condition for a child being effective in using public services and as a measure of the impact of those public services, has risen up the agenda as a result.

The approach to wellbeing amongst young people is more equivocal than that with children. Although 'children's' rights and entitlements increasingly extend to 18 or even 25 years of age, young people, like adults, are more likely to be seen as part architects of their own ill-being. They are also more likely to be seen as a threat to the wellbeing of others. Societies struggle to identify the point at which children cease to be seen as the victims of exploitation or neglect – deserving of state intervention to ensure their wellbeing both now and in the future, and become young people, increasingly responsible for their own wellbeing and potentially dangerous to themselves and others – requiring sanctions to protect the wider society from their behaviour.

Bibliography

Aries, P. (1962) *Centuries of Childhood: A Social History of Family Life*. New York.

Bacon, N., Brophy, M. Mguni, N., Mulgan, G. and Shandro, A. (2010) *The State of Happiness: Can Public Policy Shape People's Wellbeing and Resilience?* London: Young Foundation.

Batty, D. (2009) 'Timeline: A History of Child Protection'. Available at http://www.guardian.co.uk/society/2005/may/18/childrensservices2.

Beck, U. (1992) *Risk Society: Towards a New Modernity*. London: Sage.

Bessant, J. and Watts, R. (2007) *Sociology Australia*. Australia: Allan & Unwin. See http://www.allenandunwin.com/sociologyaustralia/files/RETHINK.PDF.

Bivand, P. (2003) 'What Happens to 16–18s?', Working Brief 143. London: Centre for Economic and Social Inclusion.

Bradshaw, J. and Mayhew, E. (2006) *Well-being of Children in the UK*, 2nd edn. York: York University, Social Policy Research Unit, commissioned by the Save the Children Fund.

Carter, M. (1966) *Into Work*. Harmondsworth: Penguin.

Catan, L. (2004) *Becoming Adult: Changing Youth Transitions in the 21st Century. A Synthesis of Findings from the ESRC's Research Programme – Youth, Citizenship and Social Change 1988–2003*. Brighton: Trust for the Study of Adolescence.

Children's Society (no date) 'Well-Being Monitor'. Available at http://www.childrens society.org.uk/all_about_us/what_we_do/Well-being/about_us/19908.asp.

Corsaro, W.A. (2005) *The Sociology of Childhood*. Thousand Oaks, CA: Sage.

CPAG (2009) 'Child Wellbeing and Child Poverty: Where the UK stands in the European Table'. London: Child Poverty Action Group.

Croke, R. and Crowley, A. (2007) *Stop Look and Listen: The Road to Realising Children's Rights in Wales*. Cardiff: Save the Children.

Desforges, C., with Abouchaar, A. (2003) 'The Impact of Parental Involvement, Parental Support and Family Education on Pupil Achievement and Adjustment: A Literature Review', Research Report 433. London: DfES.

Duncan, S., and Edwards, R. and Alexander, C. (eds) (2010) *Teenage Parenthood: What's the Problem?* London: Tufnell Press.

Economist (2010) 'Through a Glass Darkly', 4 February.

Feinstein, L., Hearn, B. and Renton, Z., with Abrahams, A. and MacLeod, M. (2007) *Reducing Inequalities: Realising the Talents of All*. London: National Children's Bureau.

Finch, L. (ed.) (1993) 'On the Streets: Working Class Youth Culture in the Nineteenth Century', in R. White (ed.), *Youth Subculture: Theory, History and the Australian Experience*. Hobart: National Clearinghouse for Youth Studies: 75–9.

Furlong, A. and Cartmel, F. (1997) *Young People and Social Change – Individualization and Risk in Late Modernity*. Buckingham: Open University.

Furlong, A. and Cartmel, F. (2005) *Graduates from Disadvantaged Families: Early Labour-Market Experiences*. Bristol: Policy Press.

Gangl, M. (2002) 'Changing Labour Markets and Early Career Outcomes: Labour Market Entry in Europe over the Past Decade', *Work, Employment and Society*, 16(1): 67–90.

Giddens, A. (1991) *Modernity and Self-Identity: Self and Society in the Late Modern Age*. Cambridge: Polity Press

Giddens, A. (1999) *The Third Way*. Cambridge: Polity Press.

Goleman, D. (1995) *Emotional Intelligence: Why It Can Matter More Than IQ*. New York: Bantam.

Green, A.E., Maguire, M. and Canny, A. (2001) *Keeping Track: Mapping and Tracking Vulnerable Young People*. Bristol: Policy Press.

Hagell, A. (2010) 'Time Trends in Adolescent Well-Being'. London: Nuffield Foundation.

Herford, M.E.M. (1957) *Youth at Work: A Five Year Study by an Appointed Factory Doctor*. London: Max Parrish.

Heywood, C. (2001) *A History of Childhood: Children and Childhood in the West from Medieval to Modern Times*. Cambridge: Polity Press.

Hodgson, A. (1999) 'Analysing Education and Training Policies for Tackling Social Exclusion', in A. Hayton (ed.), *Tackling Disaffection and Social Exclusion*. London: Kogan Page.

HM Treasury (2007) 'Policy Review of Children and Young People: A Discussion Paper'. London: HM Treasury.

Jones, G. (2005) *The Thinking and Behaviour of Young Adults, Literature Review for the Social Exclusion Unit*. London: Office of the Deputy Prime Minister.

Katz, I., Corlyon, J., La Placa, V. and Hunter, S. (2007) *The Relationship between Poverty and Parenting*. York: JRF.

Kay, E. (1909 [1900]) *The Century of the Child, Volume 1*. New York: Putnam.

Kennedy, D. (2006) Changing Conceptions of the Child from Renaissance to Post-Modernity: A Philosophy of Childhood. New York: Edwin Mellen Press.

Kenway, P., Parsons, N., Carr, J. and Palmer, G. (2005) *Monitoring Poverty and Social Exclusion in Wales 2005*. York: JRF.

Kohlberg, L. and Gilligan, C. (1971) 'The Adolescent as a Philosopher: The Discovery of the Self in a Postconventional World', *Daedalus*, 100(4), Fall, 1971.

Land, K.C., Lamb, V.L., Meadows, S.O. and Taylor, A. (2006) 'Measuring Trends in Child Wellbeing: An Evidence-Based Approach', International Sociological Association, Durban, South Africa.

Layard, R. and Dunn, J. (2009) *The Good Childhood Inquiry – Searching for Values in a Competitive Age*. London: Children's Society. See http://www.childrenssociety. org.uk/all_about_us/how_we_do_it/the_good_childhood_inquiry/1818.html.

Leitch, S. (2007) 'Prosperity for All in the Global Economy: World Class Skills'. London: HM Treasury.

Lister, R. (2008) 'Investing in Children and Childhood: A New Welfare Policy Paradigm and its Implications', *Comparative Social Research*, 25: 383–408.

Lloyd-Jones, S. (2005) 'A Map of Transition in the South Wales Valleys', Cardiff University, Unpublished PhD Thesis.

Lupton, R. (2004) 'Schools in Disadvantaged Areas: Recognising and Raising Quality', CASE Paper 76, available online at http://sticerd.lse.ac.uk/dps/case/cp/ CASEpaper76.pdf (accessed 15 April 2007).

Lupton, R. (2005) 'Social Justice and School Improvement: Improving the Quality of Schools in the Poorest Neighbourhoods', *British Educational Research Journal*, 31(5): 589–604.

Macdonald, R. and Marsh, J. (2005) *Disconnected Youth? Growing Up in Britain's Poor Neighbourhoods*. London: Palgrave Macmillan.

Margo, J. and Dixon, M. (2006) *Freedom's Orphans: Raising Youth in a Changing World*. London: Institute for Public Policy Research.

Milner, M. Jr. (2004) *Freaks, Geeks, and Cool Kids: American Teenagers, Schools, and the Culture of Consumption*. (New York: Routledge).

Murray, C. (1990) *The Emerging British Underclass*. London: Institute of Economic Affairs.

OECD (2009) 'Doing Better for Children'. Available at http://www.oecd.org/ document/49/0,3343,en_2649_37419_43584658_1_1_1_1,00.html.

Piaget, J. (1972) 'Intellectual Evolution from Adolescence to Adulthood', *Human Development*, 15(1): 1–12.

Putnam, R.D. (2000) *Bowling Alone: The Collapse and Revival of American Community*. New York: Simon & Schuster.

Rees, G., Bradshaw, J., Goswami, H. and Keung, A. (2010) *Understanding Children's Well-being: A National Survey of Young People's Well-Being*. London: Children's Society.

Resilience Project (no date) Available at http://www.resilienceproject.org/#What_is_ Resilience.

Rudd, P. and Evans, K. (1998) 'Structure and Agency in Youth Transitions: Student Experiences of Vocational Further Education', *Journal of Youth Studies*, 1(1): 39–62.

Rutter, M., Moffitt, T.E. and Caspi A. (2006) 'Gene–Environment Interplay and Psychopathology: Multiple Varieties but Real Effects', *Journal of Child Psychology and Psychiatry and Allied Disciplines*, 47: 226–61.

Schneider, J. (2000) 'The Increasing Financial Dependency of Young People on Their Parents', *Journal of Youth Studies*, 3(1): 3–20.

Schoon, I. (2006) *Risk and Resilience: Adaptations in Changing Times*. Cambridge: Cambridge University Press.

Tabberer, S., Hall, C., Prendergast, S. and Webster, A. (2000) *Teenage Pregnancy and Choice. Abortion or Motherhood: Influences on the Decision*. York: York Publishing Services.

UNCRC (1989) United Nation Charter on the Rights of the Child. See http://www.unicef.org.uk/pages.asp?page=92&nodeid=convent&section=2&gclid=CLj_74SVkaUCFRn-2AodnwrjLQ.

UNICEF (2007) 'Child Poverty in Perspective: An Overview of Child Well-Being in Rich Countries', *Innocenti Report Card* 7. Florence: UNICEF Innocenti Research Centre.

Welsh Assembly Government (2008) 'Children and Young People's Wellbeing Monitor'. Cardiff: Welsh Assembly Government.

Wilkinson, R. and Pickett, K. (2009) *The Spirit Level*. London: Penguin.

Williamson, H. (1997) 'Is There an Emerging British Underclass? The Evidence from Youth Research', in R. Macdonald (ed.), *Youth, The 'Underclass' and Social Exclusion*. London: Routledge: 39–54.

Wellbeing and Older People

6

Marie John

This chapter explores the concept of wellbeing in relation to older people, the challenges faced by them and those faced by society from their growing numbers. The demographic changes and the response of policy and strategy to the negative stereotyping of this age group will be outlined. Stereotyping, ageism and societal perceptions are explored from the perspectives of different sociological theories. The particular factors that affect the wellbeing of older people are discussed with some insights into physical ageing.

Definition of the older person

When the older person label should be used has been challenged and debated by society now that people are living longer in retirement. Goldman Sachs, in a global economic paper, defined age 60 as the new 55 in terms of retirement, life expectancy and economic expectations (Heacock *et al.*, 2005).

The definition of an older or elderly person proposed by the World Health Organization (WHO) suggests that most developed world countries have accepted the chronological age of 65 years as a benchmark. The WHO generally refers to persons of 60+ years as the older population (WHO, no date).

The definition is also applied to those who retire from the labour market and take their retirement pension from the state or an occupational pension from their employer. However, in times of high unemployment retirement may be offered to workers as young as 50 years. Conversely, in many instances people carry on working past the default retirement age of 65 years. Government policy is implementing a gradual equalization of the pensionable age for women from 60 to 65, the same as for men. The 10-year period for the introduction of this change will commence April 2010 (HM Government, no date). Legislation to change the default age of retirement was passed by the UK government in April 2011 (Pensions Bill, 2011). There is a short transitional period until October 2011.

The Welsh Assembly Government used 50 years and over as the benchmark for the Strategy for Older People in Wales (2003–08). This new benchmark was the subject of debate (Welsh Assembly Government, 2003).The UK National Service Framework for Older People did not specify an age, but did list services as being accessible for certain age groups such as eye tests for the over-60s and flu vaccinations for the over-65s (Department of Health, 2001). Retirement is a rite of passage that seems to signal the start of old age and is often not based on the capability of the employee to do the job but, rather, on the chronological age of the individual. Politicians, for example, seem to be outside the age parameters that apply to those for whom they legislate, and many prime ministers over the last one hundred years have been past retirement age. The retirement age of those who have economic power, a special talent or are self-employed seems to be more a matter of personal choice than a dictate of government policy.

The 'young old' 65–74, the 'old' 74–84, the 'oldest-old' 85+

Many statistics in the past divided the population into two groups: those aged below 65, and those aged over 65 (Bayliss and Sly, 2010). The population of the United Kingdom is ageing and this is projected to continue. Government statistics show that over the past 25 years the percentage of the population aged over 65 years increased from 15 per cent in 1984 to 18 per cent in 2009 – an increase of 1.7 million people. The forecast for 2034 is that 23 per cent of the population will be aged over 65 years.

The fastest increase has been in the number of those aged 85 and over, the 'oldest old'. Since 1984, the number has doubled from 660,000 to 1.4 million in 2009. By 2034, the projection is that those aged over 85 years will number 3.5 million, accounting for 5 per cent of the population (www.statistics.gov.uk). An American website that conducts research for commercial purposes divides older people into three bandings: the 'young old', aged between 65 and 74 years; the 'old', aged between 74 and 84; and the 'oldest old', aged 85 years and over (www.transgenerational.org).

The definition of the older person can be viewed in different ways depending on the context. Biological ageing to do with the changes the body undergoes is a more concrete platform but is not a uniform process for all people. Also, the rate is affected by physiological, social and psychological determinants. The influence of our genes and the way life is lived from the very earliest age has an impact on life expectancy and the degree of health and wellbeing enjoyed in later life. A health and wellbeing approach for the older generation will focus on the need to support choices that promote independent living and active engagement with society. Chronological age will not be a main facet of a wellbeing approach.

Demography of ageing

The past two hundred years have changed the population profile with the longevity of the population increasing and a gradual decrease in birth rate. However, the demographic changes across the globe are not uniform, with the developed world predicted to have 30 per cent of the population aged over 60 years by 2050. The pattern of ageing within the UK is not uniform. Wales has an older profile than England and there are regional variations, as illustrated in Figure 6.1. Northern Ireland shows the steepest projected rise for men aged over 65, and the rise for women is also high.

Less developed countries will have a lower percentage of older people in the population, making up about 20 per cent. These changes are not new and had been highlighted over fifty years ago by the United Nations (1956) The most important recent demographic change is the growth in the 'over-80s'. This change in the 'old old' has implications for all of society. This is well-illustrated by the rise in the greetings sent by the Sovereign, initially in telegram form and now in card form.

In 1917, when King George V first sent congratulations to citizens on their one hundredth birthday, he sent out 24 telegrams. In 1952, the first year of her reign, Queen Elizabeth II sent 3,000 telegrams; in 2007, she sent 8,500 cards; and, by 2031, it is projected that the number will be 40,000 (www.royal.gov.uk).

This ageing profile emphasizes the need for health and wellbeing to be central policy and practice for older people, in order to preserve the independence of this group. One way of segmenting the over-65s because of the increasing numbers is to classify those aged between 65 and 74 as the 'young old', those aged between 74 and 84 as the 'old', and those aged over 85 years as the 'oldest old'.

The current debate on changing the time when pensions are paid is conducted in the light of increasing longevity, and in an effort to reduce the financial outlay involved in paying a pension for a longer life span following retirement. The chronological definition of age has the potential to distort how health and wellbeing is viewed. Health and wellbeing promotion should be incorporated into the agenda for all policies at all levels, from local to national and international. This aspect is challenging to policymakers, but discussions of wellbeing for older people must be underpinned by the fact that the determinants of health are central to any efforts to promote health and wellbeing. The economic, social, cultural and environmental determinants and the physical aspects that are core to health and wellbeing promotion apply at all ages, but the potential for inequality and unfairness, as Black (1980) described, is a particular danger for the older person. The factors that affect older people's wellbeing include not just the visible physical changes that may affect daily functioning, but also loss of social standing, meaning and purpose, together with the possibility of loneliness, isolation and a decrease in income. These physical, psychological, emotional and social factors will be outlined but are difficult to disaggregate, as elements are interrelated and each affects the other in the experience of living. They will therefore be considered under an inclusive heading of 'ageing'.

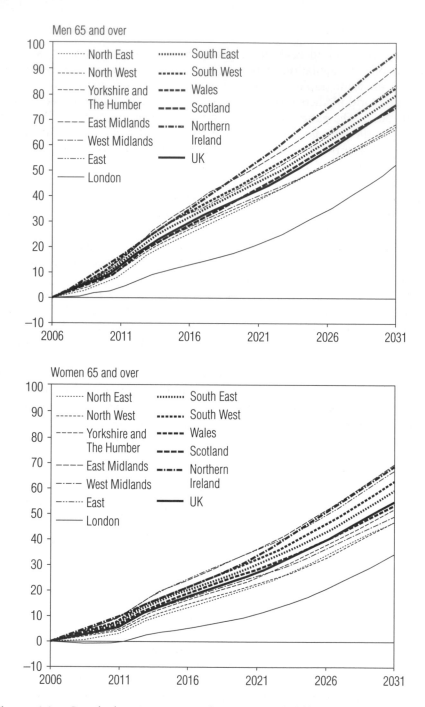

Figure 6.1 Graph showing projected UK regional differences in demographic changes in older people (2006–31)

Source: From Bayliss and Sly (2010), Office for National Statistics licensed under the Open Government Licence v.1.0.

Ageing

Understanding of the ageing process has resulted in a more fluid view of it; Kirkwood (2005) refers to ageing as 'malleable', which makes a wellbeing approach – which could improve quality of life – more desirable. Challenging the view that there is a genetic ceiling to life expectancy (Oeppens and Vaupel, 2002) presents society with the potential to use greater efforts to improve how physical ageing is experienced.

Visible evidence of the passage of years is manifested by factors such as a stooped frame, arthritic joints, hair loss, change in hair colour and the loss of skin elasticity. The loss of hearing acuity and sight, decreasing competence, and a rise in the incidence of falls and fractures are known to be linked to increasing years (Saxon et al., 2010). Manifestations of age-related changes may have an effect on the way the older person is able to live independently.

There are many negative views of the loss of function in relation to memory and ability to cope, but there is a wide spectrum of the degree to which these are a problem. The range is from mild forgetfulness and, at the other extreme, confusion and senility. In terms of health and wellbeing, there is an increasing emphasis on the value of exercise in preserving brain function. Activities that involve some intellectual challenge prove beneficial – for example, a crossword, learning a language, or doing a suduko puzzle (Hartman-Stein and Potkanowicz, 2003). The need also to feel useful and engaged and to have some control of the way life is organized and lived is an important part of feeling good about oneself. The term 'empowerment' is often used in relation to health and wellbeing (Shearer et al., 2010), and the need to feel in control and have a purpose and value will combat the negativity that society and the media attach to the older citizen. Isolation and depression with the loss of contemporary companions can result in a loss of confidence and an unwillingness to engage with their community. The need to feel valued and challenged, which may have been linked to working, will need to be replaced by other sources of personal satisfaction that promote feelings of wellbeing. For retirees who have found their work unsatisfying and stressful, the release from this way of life may result in the ability to pursue new interests and hobbies that contribute to a greater experience of wellbeing and life satisfaction. There are factors that have the potential to undermine the experience of retirement and these include physical health problems. Poverty and inequality for the older person will be linked to the loss of economic and social power, and the degree to which it is experienced is dependent on status and income prior to leaving the workforce.

Factors that affect the wellbeing of older people

The Black Report (1980) was a watershed publication that presented data to demonstrate that poverty linked to life circumstances was the main determinant of a healthy life. The evidence to support the importance of the determinants of health was presented under the sociological categories of artefact, social selection, cultural, behavioural, structuralist, and materialist.

Artefact is an explanation of how the statistics are presented and collated, which can distort the evidence. For example, the recording of occupation on death certificates can be imprecise and not accurately reflect the person's lifetime occupation. *Social selection* is concerned with movement up or down the social scale and will not be a major consideration for the older person's wellbeing. *Culture* refers to the fact that the older person will be well-established in their pattern of life, and *behavioural* change to improve health may be more difficult to achieve. *Structuralist* factors are related to how society is organized or structured and are factors that may be detrimental to wellbeing; *materialist* factors are concerned with income and standard of living. Material factors for the retired person will depend on their pension and income payments, and these are linked to occupational status prior to leaving the workplace.

The present way that society is organized, with the dominance of a market model, fails at times to recognize the contribution of the older person to society, as they are portrayed as a financial burden for those in work. This may have a negative impact, as the need to be valued and respected is important for wellbeing. The 'constellation of disadvantage' referred to in the Black Report (1980) in relation to children is equally applicable to this age group. The wealthy older person will therefore have a different experience of retirement, having an income that enables them to enjoy a higher quality of life. Poverty is an overarching health determinant, as it influences the ability to live in a pleasant locality with access to local amenities, to eat a nutritious diet, heat the home, travel at home or abroad, and employ help if necessary. Poverty will add to the worry and stress of the day-to-day life of the older person, and adversely affect their wellbeing and quality of life. Life on an occupational pension will be linked to the level of earning in employment. The state pension, on the other hand, offers only a minimum payment.

Many older people on fixed incomes can be disproportionately affected by inflation in the economy. Those with savings will be adversely affected by a drop in the interest rate, which reduces the income from investments. They comprise a vulnerable group in terms of the power they are able to exercise in the context of their own life and in the influence they exert in society. Personal power to influence circumstances of living and to engage socially is often associated with material wealth, and enjoyment of leisure activities and services depends on resources available. A contemporary perspective on inequality is offered by Wilkinson and Pickett (2010) and applies to older people who experience inequality: 'understanding the effects of inequality means that whole societies suddenly have a policy handle on the wellbeing of whole societies' (Wilkinson and Pickett, 2010: 33). Clifton (2009) also expresses the need for a new approach to the wellbeing of this growing segment of the population: 'Targeting relationships and social ties will be central to improving older people's well-being, even in the presence of other barriers to their quality of life. This will require the State to embrace a different philosophy moving away from centralized programmes that deliver a service in isolation, towards enabling and harnessing "everyday relationships".'

Wellbeing for the older person is dependent in retirement on the foundations laid over the life course. Material resources will impact on their enjoyment of life, as will their physical status. Manual work over a lifetime may result in health challenges to the individual. The body's systems for all – both rich and poor – become less efficient with age and the reserves of the human being are much reduced. Physical deficits will challenge the experience of wellbeing.

Housing and wellbeing

The factors that support health and wellbeing in older people are the same as at any other age but some factors have increased relevance; for example, housing. A reduced income and an older house with high repair bills and poor insulation may be a problem. The type of housing may also change, with retirement or sheltered housing being a preferred option for those who live alone and are in need of some minimal support. There has been an increased provision of such accommodation in the private sector, with a warden facility on site and an alert system in each flat to call for help. These flats often provide shared facilities such as a laundry and a communal sitting room, but do charge an annual fee for the facilities that are provided. Such flats are at the upper end of the market in terms of buying or renting, and this has the potential to make this type of provision unaffordable for those on a lower income, creating an inequality in housing options. In terms of wellbeing, the shared provision will afford opportunities for meeting people and mutual support.

A report in 2002 highlighted that the majority of older people live in general housing and that this requires developers to design environments around their needs and not around the service providers' needs. As the number of older people increases, their needs should be taken into account and form part of the planning and design process in new housing developments (Appleton, 2002). For example, pavements of sufficient width to cope with a wheelchair, housing door frames of the required width to use a walking frame or wheelchair and, of course, local amenities as part of the development.

Retirement villages in this country are generally found in the south of England, and aim to provide a supportive, sociable community with home ownership. The benefits are presented as 'your own front door' with privacy, security and facilities on site such as restaurants, swimming pools, and book and bowling clubs. They are mostly provided by the private sector.

Gated communities, on the other hand, are for all ages and comprise walled or fenced housing estates with closed circuit television surveillance to restrict public access to the enclosure. In practice, it seems that families tend not to choose this type of provision, but the residents are usually young professionals or retirees who are wealthy. A research study from Glasgow and Sheffield Hallam University (Atkinson et al., 2003) reported that gated communities where chosen by 80 per cent of people who had an ongoing security problem. In the report, the authors also raised the possibility that such communities had the potential to increase conflict with neighbours and the possibly that occupiers may seek to opt out of services and local taxation. There are drawbacks if older citizens are isolated from the general community as a whole, in terms of the lack of integration and potential for support from younger residents.

Brockenhurst – a village in the New Forest near Southampton, in the South of England – has a high proportion of older residents. The local general practitioner realized that patients in his surgery needed social support and opportunities for engaging in local activities. Dr Derek Browne (1995) used the WHO's 'settings approach' and an appraisal of the community, and, with pilot project funding for two years, set about 'helping the people of all ages to improve their health and wellbeing'. Partnerships with non-health partners together with a focus on participation and involvement ensured that the participants in the project felt more involved and in control – the essence of wellbeing. The Healthy Settings approach supports health and social needs, and shares a holistic view of health in common with the ideas of the Peckham Pioneer Health Centre, described in Chapter 1.

Social isolation can be a reality for the older person, especially if they have lost their partner and have no family support in the area. Some housing options have the potential to provide companionship and support but are generally only available to the wealthy, and thus can be part of increasing inequality for the older person. Loneliness can be deepened if the elderly have a physical infirmity or a loss of hearing or sight. Level of income, hobbies and interests plus membership of a church community can all be factors in whether or not social isolation is experienced.

The importance of 'place' is a theme of recent research around the older adult, and the familiarity of well-known surroundings and time lived in a place are suggested as significant to wellbeing (Rowles and Chaudhury, 2005). Local shops contribute to wellbeing and independence by providing the opportunity to choose and buy food, and to meet and talk to people. In a study conducted between 2001 and 2003, Godfrey et al. (2004) found that the localities in which people lived were of increasing importance as boundaries became more constrained.

The Young Foundation Report (Bacon et al., 2008) recommends that future policy should consider co-housing, where people could live collectively. It proposes that there should also be attention to housing and neighbourhood facilities, and that the design should facilitate the development of networks across and between the generations. The thesis is that the current emphasis on re-enablement – in terms of the physical aspects of living, evidenced by the adaptation of housing – must be extended to an emotional re-enablement.

Transport and accessibility from home have an important part to play in ensuring wellbeing for the older person, and will facilitate their involvement in social activities. In 2010, Liverpool launched a decade of health and wellbeing, and included five ways to make positive changes to life. They are: 'connect to people around you, be active, notice the world around you and the changing seasons, keep learning and give, for example, volunteer for your local community'. The project is for all ages but the sentiments apply equally for older people. The Foresight Project Mental Capacity and Wellbeing (2010) states that there is evidence that adopting these suggestions could add 7.5 years to lifespan.

Fear of crime and wellbeing

Fear of crime impacts on quality of life for the older person by decreasing their confidence and motivation to participate in local activities. Organizations need to work together to try and prevent anti-social behaviour against older citizens. A preventative approach involving the police, the local council and Age UK is likely to be most effective in creating a safe environment. A recent study of older people by the Young Foundation (Mulgan *et al.*, 2009: 157) highlighted the fear and isolation experienced by older people in society. The Young Foundation has developed an approach to community wellbeing using an assessment tool known by the acronym WARM, which stands for Wellbeing and Resilience Measure (Mguni and Bacon, 2010). This strategy could be useful for highlighting the needs of the older person in relation to their safety in the community.

Fear of crime is likely to have a detrimental effect on the wellbeing of the older person and prevent them from leaving their home, especially when it is dark. Adequate provision and maintenance of street lighting will make the outdoor environment less threatening. In addition to this, advice to older people about identity checks for all tradesmen will decrease the risk to them in their own home. The presence of policemen 'on the beat' will provide added reassurance. A survey conducted by Age Concern (now Age UK) 'The Fear Factor: Older People and Fear of Street Crime' (Boyo and Ray, 2003) found that '47% of those over 75 years of age and 37% of those over 50 no longer take part in social and community activities after dark because of fear of street crime'. A further 43 per cent of over-60s feel very or a bit unsafe walking alone after dark, 10 per cent say their life is significantly affected by fear of crime: that means over one million senior citizens (Help the Aged, 2006).

This prevalent fear runs counter to the evidence in the British Crime Survey (Flatley *et al.*, 2010), which found that the over-60s were the group least likely to be the victims of crime. The loss to the wider community if older people do not engage in volunteering activities, and to the individual from loss of the feeling of self-worth that being part of community life bestows, will have significant implications for community and individual wellbeing.

Income and the older person

The level of income for some older people has a detrimental effect on their wellbeing, although writers such as Layard (2005) and Wilkinson (1996) have proposed that it is relative income in comparison with others that has the greatest impact on health and wellbeing. Easterlin (1995) also proposed that, if basic needs are met, increased economic growth has not been shown to increase happiness. His work also shows that money does not bring happiness and talks of comparison of life circumstances with others as a major factor in life satisfaction.

The Young Foundation Report (Bacon *et al.*, 2008), in discussing low levels of life satisfaction for the older generation, states that 'if you are old and isolated and living in unfit housing or a rundown neighbourhood, worse still if you are a carer or in a care home', you will not enjoy the same level of satisfaction and, thus, wellbeing. These poor conditions for living are linked to income and to the lack of power the older person may be able to exert. Underpinning all discussions related to wellbeing and age is the importance of social support and the feeling of being involved. Bacon *et al.* (2008) state 'independence is not necessarily about the absence of help and support but an ability to make choices'. He stresses again the part played by social relationships.

Fuel poverty and older people

Fuel poverty is defined as spending at least 10 per cent of your income on heating bills. The older person is in their home for most of the day and so heating costs will be higher than average. In 2004, the Welsh Assembly Government found that 41 per cent of fuel poor households were single pensioners and 17 per cent per cent were married couples (Welsh Assembly Government, 2010).The effect on wellbeing of feeling cold is evident, but there are negative health impacts that contribute to excess winter deaths (EWDs). These deaths are in addition to what would normally be expected and are measured between December and March: fuel poverty is an additional factor to cold weather, influenza and other viral infections. EWDs in countries that have prolonged cold weather, such as Russia and Scandinavian countries, are fewer than in the UK. The pattern in Wales is similar to other regions in the UK (Welsh Assembly Government, no date).

Ageism

Age is referred to as a primitive categorization of people in addition to sex and gender. The term 'primitive' is applied because it is an automatic prejudice against a group in society (Bond *et al.*, 2007). Stereotyping is a social construction that ignores individual differences and applies group norms and values. Bytheway (1995) questions whether a focus on chronological age can be used by policymakers as a form of social control in relation to older adults. Discrimination in relation to older people is referred to as 'ageism', and is defined by the WHO as 'any distinction, exclusion or preference that has the effect of nullifying or impairing equal enjoyment of rights' (WPA/WHO, 2002).

Dependency is part of this stereotyping, and has the potential to categorize the older person as similar to a child – and consequently unable to live independently. The dependency label is often used by health and social services as a way of assessing and describing needs (Ryan *et al.*, 2006). In economic terms, there are dependency ratios that compare the economically inactive with those seen as contributing to the economy (Bond *et al.*, 2007). The relative size of the two groups as the population of older people grows has resulted in a very negative view of older people as a financial drain on those in work. This view, presented by the media, has the potential to have an adverse effect on the retired population, damaging their sense of self-worth and, thus, their wellbeing.

Data from the United Nations has drawn attention to the 'Swelling Aging Population' in a global context and describes this as a recent phenomenon). The United Nations predicts that the present 21 per cent of the population aged 60 years or over, in developed regions, may rise to 33 per cent in 2050. The rate of growth of the over-80s is projected to show the biggest change, with an almost fourfold increase by 2050 (www.un.org).

It is clear that the beginning of the twenty-first century has brought a steady increase in the age of the population after a fairly stable period towards the end of the twentieth century.

Sociology of age

There has been a general ageing of the population throughout the twentieth century, with increasing life spans for men and women (Department of Health, 2008). This has also resulted in an increase in degenerative diseases as the body ages, but this process is not inevitable and more research is needed to capture the factors that maintain good health. The present numbers of older people in the developed world is a challenge in terms of their dependence on state benefits and retirement pensions, paid out of taxation. In the less industrialized countries, there is a different demographic profile with more young people and fewer adults in the older age groups. The Western world also differs in terms of sex distribution in the population, as women live longer than men. According to the Department of Health (2008), the average age is 83 years for women and 79 years for men. Theories of ageing do not comment on this difference and most explanations are proposed from a biological perspective. Sociologists have studied the effects of ageing for the last fifty years and have attached labels to theories related to ageing. The study of sociological concepts develops an understanding of what factors affect the experience of wellbeing in older people. Three of these concepts will be outlined: disengagement theory, activity theory and continuity theory. All three seek to explain the relationship between ageing and society, and have been selected as they seem to link to the underpinnings of a wellbeing approach, with the emphasis on the elderly remaining involved, engaged and empowered within their own life as an antidote to the ageing process.

Disengagement theory suggests that older people withdraw from society and retire from work, creating opportunities for younger people to move into more responsible positions and allowing new workers to join the workforce. This disengagement has the potential to allow older people to pursue their lifetime ambitions and have greater leisure in which to enjoy their hobbies. This is a positive view and retirees with this perspective will augment their sense of wellbeing (Clarke, 2010). The converse can happen, however, with the individual becoming isolated from friends and colleagues and the social good of the workplace.

Activity theory argues that there should not be an obligation to withdraw from employment until illness makes it necessary to step down. Chronological age should not be the watershed but, rather, inability to do the job. Control is therefore given to the individual unless ill health intervenes. The fear that a loss of role within society could lead to social isolation is acknowledged, but there is a belief that new roles will have been anticipated and prepared for: Clarke calls this 'anticipatory socialisation' (Clarke, 2010).

Recent policy debates in the UK have blurred the default retirement age, and there is a gradual move to pay benefits later. However, in practice, in paid employment there is still an incentive to discontinue employment for the older person, who is often on the top of the salary scale. The wellbeing of the individual who enjoys their work would be well served by having control of their retirement timetable.

Continuity theory argues that peoples' attitudes, habits and values are fairly stable by the time they reach their later years, and their way of living established in a way that hopefully supports their wellbeing (Bond and Corner, 2004). Individuals who have developed ways of coping with life and adapting to new situations can use these skills to manage the changes that will occur as they get older. The experience of wellbeing will most likely be experienced by this latter group who have, throughout their life, coped with change. They have life skills that make the enjoyment of the new opportunities a real possibility and, if self-control and empowerment has contributed to a health enhancing lifestyle, they will have the physical capacity to enjoy their leisure (Biggs, 2007).

The three theories have been challenged as reflecting a different age, and ignoring issues of power and inequality in society (Bowling, 2005). Marmot *et al.* (2003) also support the idea that the level of engagement in society is related to social position.

The *Social System Theory* of ageing, such as the social exchange theory, modernization theory and age stratification are posited as being more appropriate, as they reflect the economic and political factors that underpin inequality. Putnam (2002) points out that no theory reflects all the areas of concern. Social exchange theory links with the level of power the individual has in the community, and suggests that older people have fewer resources to contribute – thus becoming compliant and striving to fit in and not make demands. This links to the modernization theory, as the new levels of education and technology have devalued the wisdom and skills of the older citizen. Age stratification proposes that, with age, people move to undertake different roles and younger people take their place (Bowling, 2005).

A *Salutogenic Model* proposed by Aaron Antonovsky (1979), an American sociologist, is a way of looking at life and health that is positive and opposite to *pathogenesis*, which focuses on disease and ill health. The idea of salutogenesis is that the causes of health and wellbeing should be discovered and the focus moved to how health is created, rather than how disease is prevented. The 'Sense of Coherence' is part of this life course approach and seeks to explain how people deal with stress. A global feeling of confidence, combined with comprehensibility, manageability and meaningfulness, was also part of the theory (Baker *et al.*, 2010). This enables a positive health outcome as the individual has the motivation to manage life challenges. This has links with the wellbeing movement and to the work in the 1930s of Williamson and Pearse of the Peckham Pioneer Health Centre when, although they studied the users of the centre from a disease avoidance perspective, they collected data and created an environment that supported health (Williamson and Pearse, 1966).

Societal attitudes to ageing

Attitudes are closely linked to the way the older person is viewed in a particular cultural setting – in some societies, age is equated with wisdom and the older person is given respect and status within their community. The quality of life of older people has been the subject of recent research and positive findings have resulted in a view that life can still be rewarding (Vaillant, 2002). The growth of the market economy and increasing materialism has resulted in age-related issues being viewed through the prism of an economic evaluation. The contribution of the older person and their value, if measured in terms of their output, is likely to result in a view that ignores other considerations (Meadows and Cook, 2005). The present debate about the imbalance between the growing number of older people and the numbers in the workforce who will have to support them is an example of a social attitude that is grounded in the utility of this group. The level of unpaid child care and support to working families that this group represents is often ignored. Lee (2006) comments that involvement in childcare gives older people a sense purpose and the Prime Minister's Strategy Unit (2008) reported that 26 per cent of all such provision is from this source. Their valuable contribution of £3.9 billion to the national economy and the lives of children is also significant (Lee, 2006). Participation in civil organizations represents a social good and the contribution of the older person is evident in terms of voluntary work in the community (Allen, 2008). In terms of wellbeing, this engagement with family and the wider neighbourhood is likely not only to have a positive effect on the quality of life of the retiree, but also enhance society. Material resources will impact on how engaged the person can be in terms of their ability to travel to social occasions, or pay for the cost of a ticket for the theatre or cinema. In this respect, the free bus pass makes an essential contribution to the social wellbeing of older people in providing the means of engaging in activities without the cost of travel being a factor.

Ageing and spirituality

The meaning and purpose in the older person's life may have a foundation in a religious faith that helps to explain the goal of living. Islam, for example, professes to be a way of life that presents a 'cradle to grave' philosophy, uniting its followers in a common understanding. This offers mutual support to those who share the beliefs. To a greater or lesser degree, depending on the depth of religious faith, Christian religions provide support and comfort to the older person (Millard, 2009). Spirituality is part of all people, but may manifest itself in different ways that are not necessarily concerned with religion. For example, a love of nature has a spiritual dimension for many and helps them make sense of the world. Emmons et al. (1998) conducted quality of life research and reported that personal goals that had religious or spiritual content had an important influence on wellbeing. The strength that is offered by a view of life after death, which forms part of many religious faiths, helps individuals to have a positive vision of the future. Church, synagogue, temple and mosque offer a social centre for communal prayer and mutual support for shared values and beliefs. Many of these places of worship also augment social provision in the community through local groups, from luncheon clubs to flower arranging and coach trips. Spirituality can be separate from religious association, but both qualities have the potential to promote the wellbeing of the older person.

A study by Wilkinson and Coleman (2010) tested the view that a belief system acted as a coping mechanism for older people, helping them to manage stress and loss. They matched two groups of over-60s who had experienced similar losses, both of which had a strong belief system. They concluded it was the strength of the belief system – not whether or not it was religious or atheistic – that helped and, thus, provided explanation, consolation, support and inspiration for the interviewees living in southern England.

Conclusion

O'Sullivan and Mulgan (2010), in a paper published through the Young Foundation, propose the need for social innovation in ageing societies and sum up the way forward:

> Innovation in this context sees older people not as a burden but as a valuable resource: it enables their contribution, seeing them as active participants and not passive consumers; and it focuses on capabilities as well as needs. Underpinning all of this is a focus on improving the quality of life for older people, emphasizing a shift away from an exclusive focus on health and pensions to more holistic focus on wellbeing.

Wellbeing, therefore, as a goal for policy and practice, has contemporary resonance as it is a non-age-related concept and encompasses the needs of the older person within a societal framework. The role of the older person as a contributor to the 'Big Society' needs to be valued, and even expanded. The centrality of the social world to the experience of wellbeing is a challenge to how services are planned and delivered in the future. The way forward should harness the capability of this group and engage them in activities and services to the community, thus increasing their sense of worth and wellbeing. Older people must feel valued, respected and understood in order to foster good mental health and wellbeing (Lee, 2006).

Life expectancy has increased, and the goal of policy and practice must be to maintain quality of life, independence and a sense of wellbeing – an essential component of a positive outlook of life. The term 'wellbeing' therefore has contemporary relevance as a non-age-related concept, and its attainment and continuance must be a goal for all older citizens. The life course for all people represents changes in lifestyle, economic status and physical capabilities. For the older person, the contribution they make to society and their own community may increase, despite the fact that their power to influence their own life may be less as they are on a fixed income that they cannot change. The term 'the older person' is, in itself, contentious: where does old age start; what factors define it successfully when it is so individual? The number of years of life lived is often the means of definition, but the biological age may be different from the chronological age. The much overused concept of empowerment and having control over the challenges and opportunities that are part of increasing age are vital to a sense of wellbeing. The theme of the centrality of the social world, and the need for the older person to feel engaged and part of society, has threaded through this chapter. The value of paid work as the most important source of personal satisfaction, and thus wellbeing, is an important fact that needs to be part of policy considerations. Exit from work is likely to be delayed in the future, with a resultant increase in wellbeing. The time that has elapsed since leaving the labour market affects social participation, and thus wellbeing; and, for men, wealth has a strong independent effect. For women, it is subjective social status that has the most relevance (Hyde and Jones, 2007). Higgs and Jones comment that the inequalities over the life course cast a 'long shadow' that affects social economic position and, thus, inequalities persist in retirement (Higgs and Jones, 2008). The United Nations Principles for the Older Person (adopted by the General Assembly 16/91 in December 1991) are independence, participation, care, self-fulfilment and dignity (UN, 1991). These principles chime well with the wellbeing agenda, and the goal of a more equal and inclusive role for older people within an innovative approach that not only considers entitlement and health problems, but also actively promotes positive health and wellbeing.

Bibliography

Allen, J. (2008) 'Older People and Wellbeing', in *Challenging Times: Changing Policy*. London: Institute for Public Policy Research (IPPR).

Antonovsky, A. (1979) *Health, Stress and Coping: New Perspectives on Mental and Physical Wellbeing*. New York: Jossey-Bass.

Appleton, N. (2002) *Planning for the Majority: The Needs and Aspirations of Older People in General Housing*. York, UK: Joseph Rowntree Trust.

Atkinson, R., Flint, J., Blandy, S. and Lister, D. (2003) Gated Communities in England: Final Report of the Gated Communities in England. 'New Horizons' Project, University of Glasgow and Sheffield Hallam University.

Bacon, N., Brophy, M., Mguni, N., Mulgan, G. and Shandro, A. (2008) *The State of Happiness: Can Public Policy Shape People's Wellbeing and Resilience?* London: Young Foundation.

Baker, C., Glascoff, M. and Fells, W. (2010) 'Salutogenesis 30 years Later: Where Do We Go From Here?', *International Electronic Journal of Health Education*, 13: 25–32.

Bayliss, J. and Sly, F. (2010) 'Ageing across the UK'. Office for National Statistics.

Biggs, S. (2007) 'Thinking about Generations: Conceptual Positions and Policy Implications', *Journal of Social Issues*, 63(4): 695–711(17).

Black Report (1980) *Inequalities in Health: Report of a Research Working Group*. London: DHSS

Bond, J. and Corner, L. (2004) *Quality of Life and Older People*. Buckingham: Open University Press

Bond, J., Peace, S., Dittmann-kohli, F. and Westerhoff, G. (2007) 'Ageing in Society: European Perspectives on Gerontology'. London: Sage Publications.

Bowling, A. (2005) *Ageing Well: Quality of Life in Old Age*. London Open University Press.

Boyo, S. and Ray, S. (2003) *The Fear Factor: Older People and Fear of Street Crime – A Survey of Views, Experiences and Impact on Quality of Life*. Age Concern Books. (See also http://www.ageuk.org.uk/professional-resources-home/policy)

Browne, D. (1995) Healthy Villages: Occasional Paper. Royal College of General Practitioners.

Bytheway B (1995) *Ageism*. Buckingham: Open University Press.

Clarke, A. (2010) *The Sociology of Healthcare*, 2nd edn. England: Pearson Education.

Clifton, J. (2009) 'Ageing and Wellbeing in an International Context: Politics of Ageing', *Working Paper* 3, Institute for Public Policy Research.

Community Safety NI (no date) Available at www.communitysafetyni.gov.uk.

Department for Transport (2004) *Traffic Signs Manual*, ch. 4 'Warning Signs'.

Department of Health (2001) 'Modern Standards and Service Models: Older People National Service Framework'. London: DOH.

Department of Health (2008) Life Expectancy and All Age All Cause Mortality and Monitoring (Overall and Health Inequalities): Update to include data for 2007, available at: www.dh.gov.uk/en/Publicationsandstatistics/Publications/Publications Statisitcs/DH_090133 (accessed 21 November 2010).

Emmons, R., Cheung, C. and Tehrani, K. (1998) 'Assessing Spirituality through Personal Goals: Implications for Research on Religion and Subjective Wellbeing', *Social Indicators Research*, 45: 391–422.

Easterlin, R. (1995) 'Will Raising the Incomes of All Increase the Happiness of All?', *Journal of Economic Behaviour and Organisation*, 27: 35–47.

Flatley, J., Kershaw, C., Smith, K., Chaplin, R. and Moon, D. (2010) 'Home Office Statistical Bulletin: Crime in England and Wales 2009/10'. Home Office.

Foresight for Mental and Wellbeing (2010) 'Year of Health and Wellbeing'. Available at www.2010healthandwellbeing.org.uk/index.php (accessed 28 October 2010).

Godfrey, M., Townsend, J. and Denby, T. (2004) *Building a Good Life for Older People in Local Communities. The Experience of Ageing in Time and Place*. Joseph Rowntree Foundation.

Hartman-Stein, P. and Potkanowicz, E. (2003) 'Behavioural Determinants of Healthy Aging: Good News for the Baby Boomer Generation', *Online Journal of Issues in Nursing*, 8(2): 5.

Heacock, D., Lawson, S. and Purushothaman, R. (2005) '60 Is the New 55: How the G6 Can Mitigate the Burden of Aging', *Goldman Sachs: Global Economic Paper* no. 132.

Help the Aged (2006) 'Crime and Fear of Crime', Policy Statement, available at http://www.ageuk.org.uk/documents/en-gb/forprofessionals/communities-and-inclusion/crime_and_fear_of_crime_2006_pro.pdf?dtrk=true.

Higgs, P. and Jones, I. (2008) *Medical Sociology and Old Age: Towards a Sociology of Health in Later Life*. Oxford: Routledge.

HM Government (no date) Available at www.direct.gov.uk.

Hyde, M. and Jones, I.R. (2007) 'The Long Shadow of Work: Does Time since Labour Market Exit Affect the Association between Socioeconomic Position and Health in a Post-Working Population', *Journal of Epidemiology and Community Health*, 61(6): 533.

Kirkwood, T. (2005) 'Understanding the Odd Science of Ageing', *Cell*, 120: 437–47.

Layard, R. (2005) Happiness: Lessons from a New Science. London: Penguin.

Lee, M. (2006) 'Promoting Mental Health and Well-Being in Later Life: A First Report from the UK Inquiry into Mental Health and Well-Being in Later Life'. London: Mental Health Foundation and Age Concern.

Marmot, M., Banks, J., Blundell, R., Lessof, C. and Nazroo, J. (eds) (2003) *Health, Wealth and Lifestyles of the Older Population in England: The 2002 English Longitudinal Study of Ageing.* London: Institute of Fiscal Studies.

Meadows, P. and Cook, W. (2005) 'The Economic Contribution of Older People'. London: Age Concern.

Mguni, N. and Bacon, N. (2010) *Taking the Temperature of Local Communities.* Young Foundation. Available at www.youngfoundation.org.

Millard, P. (2009) 'Book Review: *Ageing, Disability and Spirituality*', *Age and Ageing*, 38(3): 356.

Mulgan, G., Ali, R. and Norman, W. (2009) *Sinking and Swimming: Understanding Britain's Unmet Needs.* Young Foundation. Available at www.youngfoundation. org.

Oeppens, J. and Vaupel, J. (2002) 'Demography: Broken Limits to Life Expectancy', *Science*, 296: 1029–31.

O'Sullivan, C. and Mulgan, G. (2010) *Innovating Better Ways of Living in Later Life: Context, Examples and Opportunities.* Young Foundation. Available at www.youngfoundation.org (accessed 14 November 2010).

Peckham Pioneer Health Centre (no date) 'The Peckham Experiment'. Available at http://www.thephf.org/.

Pensions Bill (2011) Available at http://wwwhttp://www.thephf.org/.publications. parliament.uk/pa/bills/lbill/2010 2011/0061/11061.pdf.

'Pensions and Retirement Planning: Calculating Your State Pension'. Government's announcement to changes to state pension age. Available at http://www.direct. gov.uk/en/Pensionsandretirementplanning/StatePension/DG4017919 (accessed 4 October 2010).

Prime Minister's Strategy Unit (2008) 'Realising Britain's Potential: Future Strategic Challenges for Britain'. London: Cabinet Office.

Putnam, M. (2002) 'Linking Ageing Theory and Disability Models: Increasing the Potential to Explore Ageing with Physical Impairment', *Gerontologist*, 42: 799–806.

Rees, P. and Jones, I.R. (2008) *Medical Sociology and Old Age: Towards a Sociology of Health in Later Life.* London: Routledge.

Rowles, G. and Chaudhury, H. (eds) (2005) 'Home and Identity in Later Life', in *International Perspectives*. New York: Springer: 521–46.

Royal.gov.uk The official website of the British Monarchy. Available at http://www. royal.gov.uk/HMTheQueen/Queenandanniversarymessages/Factsandfigures.aspx.

Ryan, M., Netten, A., Skatun, D. and Smith, P. (2006) 'Using Discrete Choice Experiments to Estimate a Preference-Based Measure of Outcome: An Application to Social Care for Older People', *Journal of Health Economics*, 25(5): 927–44.

Saxon, S., Etten, M. and Perkins, E. (2010) *Physical Change and Ageing: A Guide for the Helping Professions.* New York: Springer.

Shearer, C., Nelma, B., Fleury, J. and Belyea, M. (2010) 'Randomized Control Trial of the Health Empowerment Intervention: Feasibility and Impact', *Nursing Research*, 59(3): 203–11.

United Nations (1956) 'The Aging of Populations and its Economic and Social Implications', *Population Studies* no. 26, United Nations publication, Sales No. 1956. XIII.6.

United Nations (1991) United Nations Principles for Older Persons Adopted by General Assembly resolution 46/91 of 16 December 1991. Available at http://www2.ohchr.org/english/law/olderpersons.htm (accessed 5 December 2010).

United Nations (2008) Available at www.un.org./esa/population/publications/wpp2008/wpp2008/wpp2008_highlights.pdf (accessed 2 June 2011).

United Nations (2009) 'The Swelling Aging Population. A Recent Global Phenomenon'. Available at http://www.transgenerational.org/aging/demographics.htm#Characteristics#ixzz166e2FW6v (accessed 5 December 2010).

Vaillant, G. (2002) *Ageing Well: Surprising Guideposts to a Happier Life from the Landmark Study of Adult Development*. Boston, MA: Little, Brown & Co.

Welsh Assembly Government (no date) Available at www.wales.gov.uk/statistics (accessed 12 December 2010).

Welsh Assembly Government (2003) 'The Strategy for Older people in Wales 2003–2008', Cardiff: Welsh Assembly Government.

Welsh Assembly Government (2010) Living in Wales – Fuel Poverty Statistics Welsh Assembly Government. Available at http://wales.gov.uk/docs/caecd/research/110321fuel.pdf.

Whitehead, M. (1988) *The Health Divide: Inequalities in Health in the 80s*. London: Health Education Authority.

WHO (no date) 'Definition of an Older or Elderly Person'. Available at http://www.who.int/healthinfo/survey/ageingdefnolder/en/index.html (accessed 22 November 2010).

Wilkinson, P. and Coleman, P. (2010) 'Strong Beliefs and Coping in Old Age: A Case-Based Comparison of Atheism', *Ageing and Society*, 30(2): 337–61.

Wilkinson, R. (1996) *Unhealthy Societies: The Afflictions of Inequality*. London: Routledge.

Wilkinson, R. and Pickett, K. (2010) *The Spirit Level: Why Equality is Better for Everyone*. London: Penguin.

Williamson, G. and Pearse, I. (1966) 'Science and Synthesis, and Sanity: An Inquiry into the Nature of Living', cited in C. Baker, M. Glascoff and W. Fells (2010) 'Salutogenesis 30 Years Later: Where Do We Go From Here?', *International Electronic Journal of Health Education*, 13: 25–32.

WPA (World Psychiatric Association) and WHO (World Health Organization) (2002) 'Reducing Stigma and Discrimination against Older People with Mental Disorders', Technical Consensus Statement, Geneva.

www.2010healthandwellbeing.org.uk/index.php (accessed 5 October 2010).

Wellbeing and Work

Gemma Pates

This chapter explores some of the contextual influences that have shaped the modern workplace and influenced individual experience of work, including organizational restructuring, the impact of information technology (IT), the increasing dominance of the service industries, the growing representation of women in the workforce, and the impact of the current recession. It concludes by looking at the policy reforms that these influences and experiences have necessitated, particularly in the light of the Black Report (2008).

Introduction

Since the turn of the millennium, the relationship between work and wellbeing has taken centre stage on the political agenda, and driven a fundamental rethink in UK public health and welfare policy. As work forms a significant part of life experience, it potentially has a substantial impact on our physical and psychological health – and, ultimately, our wellbeing.

In an extensive review of the literature, Waddell and Burton (2006) concluded that there is a convincing evidence base that work is good for health and wellbeing. But is it? If this is the case, how can the economic cost of sickness absence and worklessness be explained? In a review of the working age population, Dame Carol Black (2008) estimated this cost to be £100 billion annually. This figure is clearly significant in the current climate of economic downturn and a cost that the economy, employers and, indeed, individuals can ill afford to bear.

Setting the context of work: contemporary careers

The ways in which people experienced work changed dramatically during the latter part of the twentieth century. Organizations undertook extensive restructuring and downsizing in order to achieve a more flexible and efficient workforce. This resulted in flatter organizational structures with fewer hierarchical levels. In addition, increasing globalization meant that organizations were able to cut costs by off-shoring and outsourcing. While these processes resulted in organizational benefits, from an employee perspective they resulted in more intense job responsibilities and longer working hours (Brockner *et al.*, 1992). In a study of UK employees, Green (2006) suggested that the effect of such structural changes on employees is a decline in overall job satisfaction.

Furthermore, technological advances have significantly transformed working practices. Organizations have become increasingly 'virtual', characterized by computer mediated involvement in work. This has meant that for some employees the demand for direct face-to-face engagement has decreased. The effects of technological advancements are mixed; while for some it has enhanced wellbeing through improved effectiveness, for others it has resulted in de-skilling and tighter managerial control (Eason, 2002), not to mention increased risk of musculoskeletal disorders.

These developments are associated with a change in the nature of work itself. Previously dominant industries such as manufacturing and utilities have declined, whilst technical, managerial and professional work have seen marked expansion. Predictions made by the Working Futures report for 2007–17 suggest this trend is likely to persist, with the manufacturing and utilities industries continuing to diminish. The growth of the so-called service industries demonstrates the change in organizational values from physical assets to human capital, accompanied by an increasing number of individuals entering the workforce with higher-level educational qualifications.

What impact has the recession had on wellbeing? The recent recession has further added to employees' perceptions of an uncertain future and job insecurity. As may be expected, the wellbeing of workers is lower in times of recession, as is satisfaction with pay and job security. However, contrary to what might have been predicted, job satisfaction itself is higher within times of recession (Clarke, 2011).

In a further analysis of the impact of the 2008/09 recession, Faggio *et al.* (2011) find job tenure to average 10 years, which is much the same as it was in the 1980s. Whereas, on the surface, this finding appears positive, they go on to note that job tenure for men has decreased, while that for women has increased. This marks the increased representation of women in the workforce, which is perhaps due to the increasing provision of family-friendly policies designed to enable better work–life balance.

Dolton and Makepeace (2011) indicate that female workers are more likely to be in the public sector, with two thirds of that sector's workforce being female in 2008 and 2009. They also note that there appears to be a significant degree of 'sector envy' during the current recession, with private sector workers believing that public sector equivalents are better off. This may be, in part, due to the long-standing perception that the public sector was protected from budget cuts and subsequent job losses. However, this perception is beginning to change somewhat. An article by O'Dowd (2011) published in the *British Medical Journal* warned of National Health Service job cuts after failed negotiations over pay.

Some authors argue that the contemporary context of work has constrained the 'traditional' career. As organizations take on more horizontal management structures, the potential for upward mobility, seniority and corresponding remuneration has become limited. This has caused some debate on how best to conceptualize careers in contemporary work organizations.

Whilst some believe that the notion of 'career' is inextricably linked to professional work and advancement, others take a broader view. As Kidd (2002) notes, 'no one who spends any time in employment or seeking employment is excluded from having a career' (p. 179). Perhaps what is more significant is the emergence of the 'boundaryless' careers concept, which highlights the change in values towards work. Sullivan (1999) summarized the boundaryless career as one that emphasizes performance, with skills that are portable across multiple organizations, has a continuous learning philosophy and values psychologically meaningful work rather than status. Therefore, boundaryless organizations (Askenas, 1999) pay more attention to individual input, added value and tacit knowledge in achieving organizational and societal gains. As a result, investment through people has become a key priority in what has become known as the 'knowledge economy'.

It is important to consider these contextual factors in terms of the impact on employee attitudes and behaviours – and, ultimately, their wellbeing. This may depend on the extent to which employees identify with their work as part of a greater life interest or simply view it as a means to an end; 'Living to Work – Working to Live' (Guest and Sturges, 2007: 310). By definition, work has no prerequisite condition that it is to be enjoyed; rather, it is simply an activity that expends mental and/or physical effort.

So, what effect has this changing career context had on employees? Clearly, the picture is not necessarily a positive one, given the high cost of working age ill health. Intensive workloads, long working hours, low job satisfaction, reduced autonomy and higher self reported stress levels have surely had an impact on undesirable work behaviours such as absenteeism, presenteeism and overall reduced productivity. In addition, high skill levels have become favoured, and poor pension provision has meant a higher proportion of ageing workers. However, what are less clear are the exact mechanisms of influence and the extent to which the effects are moderated by other variables. This has generated substantial research interest and resulted in increased provision of services to enhance employee wellbeing within organizations. Most prominently, stress management training, occupational health access and, for the more in need, employee assistance programmes. However, many of these seem to have a preoccupation with 'fixing the sick' (Seligman, 1999).

But can work be good for health and wellbeing? The extensive review of the literature by Waddell and Burton (2006) provided a best evidence response. They found that:

- employment is an important means for obtaining material assets for engagement in society;
- work fulfils psychosocial needs;
- work defines identity, social roles and status within society; and
- employment and social economic status are factors in social differentials in physical and mental health and mortality.

However, it is noted that work can pose physical and psychosocial hazards and therefore has a potential risk to health.

Overall their conclusion is that the beneficial effects of work outweigh the risks (Waddell and Burton, 2006). This review has been pivotal in driving policy away from 'the negative legacy' approach (Fineman, 2006).

But perhaps more significant is the assertion that work can play a positive role in recovery from ill health and enhance general health and wellbeing. Waddell and Burton (2006) suggest that, for sick and disabled people, work can be therapeutic, improve health outcomes and lessen the likelihood of long-term incapacity, as well as providing financial security, promoting social participation and improving overall quality of life. Therefore, reducing long-term incapacity and working age ill health are key elements in policy reform.

Current policy: the government response to the Black Report

The Black Report (2008) notes the dominant perception that illness is incompatible with work. Therefore, the recommendations set out to remedy this preconception and advocate a more proactive approach with a clear message: 'good health is good business' (p. 54).

The review has three principle objectives:

- promoting health and wellbeing and preventing illness;
- providing early intervention for those who develop ill health; and
- improving the health of the workless, thereby increasing the potential for work.

These objectives underpin the extensive recommendations for policy reform to address not just the economic impact of working age ill health, but also to fulfil moral and social obligations to individuals, families and society in general.

Historically, there appears to have been little in the way of disease prevention and health promotion in work-based settings other than rhetoric and meeting a minimum in legal compliance, as organizations considered there to be little justification for investment beyond ensuring adequate health and safety.

However, despite individual lifestyle choices being the major cause of working age ill health, there is a growing body of evidence that there is a business case for employer investment in health and wellbeing. Kuoppala *et al.* (2008)

concluded that work-based health promotion was effective not only in improving employee wellbeing and work ability, but also in reducing sickness absence. But they note that education and psychological interventions alone were more limited in effectiveness, suggesting a need to target both physical and psychosocial aspects.

Similarly, Mills *et al.* (2007) studied the impact of health promotion programmes on employee health risks and work productivity, concluding that they yielded a positive return on investment.

The governmental response to the Black Report, *Improving Health and Work: Changing Lives* (Waddell and Burton, 2006) recognizes the need for multi-agency investment. It sets out a cross-governmental initiative to remedy the previously fragmented approach, to encourage positive communication amongst partners and to emphasize shared responsibility for promoting and maintaining health and wellbeing.

The key elements of the policy are:

- changing perceptions regarding health by introducing an electronic 'fit note' to replace the traditional 'sick note';
- providing an education programme for general practitioners to improve confidence in advising people with health conditions with regard to returning to or staying in work;
- introducing health work and wellbeing co-ordinators to take a proactive approach in promotion of wellbeing and an advisory role particularly with small and medium-sized enterprises (SMEs); and
- establishing a national centre for working age health and wellbeing as an independent body to collate data and analysis regarding effectiveness, and encourage ongoing research.

Whilst these initiatives are indicative of dramatic reform, the Governmental Response (2008) notes that some of the existing provisions such as Access to Work and NHS Plus are to remain, albeit in a modified and extended format. However, this really is just the starting point in changing practices and, ultimately, attitudes and behaviours.

As Waddell and Burton (2006) point out, work is good for wellbeing but there are three major provisos on this conclusion that represent some of the key challenges for the success of policy reform. They note that:

- the results indicate average effects and there is a minority of people for whom work may produce negative effects on health and wellbeing;
- the nature and quality of work are important moderators of the beneficial effects on health and wellbeing; and
- the social context must be taken into consideration – specifically, regional areas of deprivation.

These provisos are discussed in greater detail within the context of key target groups in policy reform (pp. 124–5).

Improving health, happiness and wellbeing

Many of the interventions that organizations offer in relation to wellbeing have been designed to address the rising problem of work-related stress. This is perhaps, in part, due to a persuasive stress management discourse that has followed the increased incidence of stress that has occurred since the 1980s. The Health and Safety Executive (HSE) define work related stress as 'the adverse reaction people have to excessive pressures or other types of demand placed on them at work'.

However, many academics believe that the widespread adoption of the stress concept has severely limited progress in the field of work and wellbeing. Indeed, there is certainly a lack of consensus with regard to establishing a clear definition of stress. This can be largely explained by different disciplines referring to stress as being both stimulus and response; that is, stress being the cause of an uncomfortable psychological state and also being the resultant state itself.

In addition, the effectiveness of stress management interventions is still unclear. Briner and Reynolds (1999) challenge the assumption that organizational stress causes lower levels of wellbeing and performance and increases absence and turnover, and that reducing stress will reverse these effects. They suggest that this is based on two unsupportable propositions: that stress causes undesirable states and behaviours, and that interventions will work with uniformly positive effects. They conclude, 'Until we know and understand the causes of negative employee states and behaviours, and know and understand how and if organizational interventions work, our interventions will continue to be simple and clear-but also hopelessly wrong' (p. 661). Despite this, work related stress is still a dominating concept in working-age ill health.

The HSE report for 2009/2010 estimates the prevalence of musculoskeletal disorders to be 572,000 and that of stress, anxiety and depression to be 435,000. These figures represent the highest cited causes of sickness-related absence. Despite the higher prevalence of musculoskeletal disorders, mental ill health has a higher resultant cost in terms of working days lost. The HSE data also indicate that personal service and associated professional/technical occupations had the highest incidences of work-related illness. This is perhaps consistent with the changing nature of work.

Therefore, it may be argued that there are high risk occupations. A study of work-related stress across occupations in the UK found ambulance workers, teachers, social services, customer services, call centres, prison officers and police to have worse than average physical and psychological wellbeing and lower job satisfaction (Johnson et al., 2005). The authors speculate that the high levels of emotional labour associated with highly stressful jobs may be a causal factor.

Possibly the most significant proviso that Waddell and Burton (2006) make is that in relation to job quality. Coats and Lekhi (2008) characterize quality jobs as secure, autonomous and discretionary, with an absence of monotony and repetition. In addition, the workplace should provide a balance between effort and reward, and foster strong workplace relationships.

There is certainly evidence that jobs with poor job quality have a negative impact on health and wellbeing. Jianli *et al.* (2010) found that job strain and effort–reward imbalance had a negative effect on job performance through the severity of the resultant depression. Therefore, they suggest work-based health promotion should target work–family conflict as well as job characteristics to reduce the risk of depression and subsequent poor job performance.

Shift work is often thought of as having a negative effect on health and wellbeing. A study of junior doctors' shift patterns found frequent on call periods increased perceptions of poor work–life balance and psychological strain (Tucker *et al.*, 2010). In addition, shift work has been associated with an increased morbidity for a number of health-related disorders such as depression, gastrointestinal and cardiovascular risks (Waterhouse *et al.*, 1992).

Similarly, call centre work has been criticized for requiring operatives to follow tight scripts, reducing the role for employee autonomy and subjecting employees to tight controls. Knights and McCabe (1998) investigated the effect of business process re-engineering (BPR) – a process designed to provide cost effective and flexible customer orientated services – on staff stress. Their findings indicated that following BPR for those staff remaining in employment, work became more intensive and stressful. Moreover, technology that may be implemented to gain tighter control over employees' work processes may be manipulated by employees in ways that are not consistent with organizational goals. This may suggest that employees act in ways to create their own diverse and autonomous roles and, simultaneously, seek to enhance their wellbeing.

However, the issue of job quality is a fairly recent issue for policy. Green (2011) suggests the key aspects of job quality are pay, work-life balance, skills, autonomy and work effort. In a review of the effect of the recession on these aspects he notes that there is still much to be done on improving job design. Green (2011) suggests that while pay, working hours and work–life balance have seen improvements, skills in terms of supply and demand are not rising fast enough, employees have less discretion, and work intensity and work stress remain prominent issues.

A finding by the Workplace Employee Relations Survey (2004) found that wellbeing is partly determined by the workplace itself, and not just by demographics or the characteristics of the job.

Unemployment

Waddell and Burton (2006) concluded that there is a significant link between unemployment and poor physical and mental health and mortality, which appears to be largely a causal relationship.

As part of an overarching reform in policy the Welfare Reform Bill (2011) sets out fundamental changes to the current benefit system, and plans to extend the revisions that have already been undertaken. The key elements of the bill are:

- rethinking incentives to work to ensure that work always pays;
- protecting the most vulnerable individuals in society; and
- ensuring fairness.

How will the bill achieve this?

The introduction of a universal credit aims to further the simplification of the benefits system and allow more opportunity to demonstrate the value of being in work. In additional, new claimant commitments will be introduced to make clear expectations from claimants at the outset, and disability related payments will be altered to ensure protection for those with the greatest needs. Further, sanctions are proposed for those who repeatedly turn down employment opportunities. Again, this marks the policy shift in the ways working age health and unemployment are being conceptualized, emphasizing what individuals can achieve rather than what they cannot.

However, critics argue that the bill may surreptitiously punish the already worse off groups in society. At the greatest risk are the unskilled and inexperienced groups with a long history of incapacity and unemployment. In addition, it is important to note that the use of sanctions will not necessarily push people into employment; rather, it may turn them to other means of securing income – for example, through criminal activity.

Gregg *et al.* (1999) found that 18 per cent of UK households with working age adults had no one in employment. This statistic still holds over a decade later (ONS, 2010). Therefore, they suggest, for a small yet notable minority of the population worklessness is their 'career'. While this can largely be attributed to a regional lack of employment opportunity, where opportunities do exist they are poorly paid and do not adequately substitute for welfare payments. This is supported by Dolton *et al.* (2011), who show that the highest proportion of minimum wage workers are in the North, the Midlands and South and West Wales. These areas would have previously been characterized by high levels of industrial employment.

If work is good for health and wellbeing, then it follows that unemployment should be to their detriment, and there is certainly a large body of evidence that supports this. But it is important to note that the effects of unemployment extend far beyond pecuniary restrictions (Winkleman, 2008). In a German study, Kassenboehmer and Haisken-DeNew (2009) demonstrated entry into unemployment had a strong negative effect on life satisfaction.

However, a longitudinal study by Lin and Leung (2010) demonstrated the differential effect of coping strategies on a sample of long-term unemployed. When job searching was the primary method of coping, this had a negative effect on mental health – largely due to situational appraisals, unemployment and economic hardship. Conversely, where emotional distancing from unemployment was the primary coping mechanism, this had a positive effect on mental health, even when situational factors were taken into account, and the positive effects were long-lasting.

The recession has also further impacted on the health of the unemployed in terms of decreased wellbeing and higher levels of depression, in addition to financial difficulties (Bell and Blanchflower, 2010). Further, Bell and

Blanchflower note that the greatest effect has been on the younger members of the working age population, with the result being increased numbers of applications for higher education within this group. However, this trend may diminish in the future due to the recent government changes that lifted the cap on tuition fees, meaning that some universities may charge up to £9000 per year. This may mean that, for some, especially for those from poorer backgrounds, education comes at too high a price.

Undoubtedly, young people represent a significant challenge for policy success. The number of unemployed aged between 16 and 24 reached 965,000 in the quarter up to December 2010. This is the highest recorded figure since records began (ONS, 2011a).

Perhaps the greatest challenges relate to the more socially deprived pockets of society where intergenerational welfare use is most prevalent. In a US study, Rank and Cheng (1995) found that children who grow up in households that receive welfare payments are more likely to become welfare claimants in adulthood. They suggest that being raised in lower-income households negatively impacts on children's development of human capital. This is of particular concern in a labour market that values human capital as a competitive advantage.

Similarly, an early UK study of unemployment trends through families suggests unemployed youth are more likely than their employed peers to have another family member who is unemployed. This implies it is a significant factor in developing attitudes of young people towards work (Payne, 1987). In addition, there is evidence to suggest that organizational restructuring has limited the opportunity for unemployed people to enter the labour force, particularly in the case of older workers (Payne and Payne, 1994). This inability to utilize skills can result in a skill depreciation effect and impaired quality of life (Ranzijn et al., 2006).

Current estimates show that approximately 8 per cent of the economically active are unemployed. But, a critical point may be whether the economy has the right kind of jobs available.

Ageing workforce

The proportion of people in the workforce aged 65 years or over has doubled over the last decade (ONS, 2011b). Therefore, as Black (2008) points out, a large proportion of time spent in poor health is likely to be experienced during working age. Whereas the parents of the baby boom generation demonstrated a trend towards early retirement, this trend has reversed, with the resultant effect being higher economic activity levels among those aged over 50 (Disney et al., 2011). This trend is sure to continue, as state pension age is to be increased for both men and women to 68 years by 2046.

The rise of the knowledge economy and boundaryless careers has called for a culture of continuous learning and development from employees in order to maintain a competitive advantage. Therefore, employees who are unable to maintain their skill levels in line with organizational demands may become obsolete (Greller and Stroh, 1995). While it may be expected that older work-ers are more susceptible to the effects of recession, Disney *et al.* (2011: 56) demonstrate that that they have, in fact, been 'relatively recession proof'.

Further, it might be expected that older workers are more likely to demon-strate absenteeism behaviours. However, Feldman (2007) notes that the reverse is true, suggesting that older workers with significant health problems are more likely to exit the labour market through retirement. However, poor pension provision means that this may not be a financially viable option for all employees. Wester and Wolff (2010) suggest that, despite attempts to reduce health inequalities, these persist. They propose that workers who are exposed to health risks by their employment should be allowed to access their state pension early, regardless of whether they choose to retire or not. The effect of this may be a phased reduction in exposure to harmful work factors (e.g. work related stress), by allowing opportunity to reduce duties or hours without jeopardizing financial security.

Conclusion

It is widely believed that the healthy and happy worker is a productive worker. However, the economic cost of working age ill health is significant and, set against a context of recession, represents an enormous challenge for policy reform. The latter part of the twenty-first century dramatically changed orga-nizational structure and function and, ultimately, the ways in which employ-ees experience work.

Human capital became our most valuable competitive advantage, and increased the general skill and educational level of the workforce. Whilst, on the surface, this appears to be a positive development, it brought with it an unfortunate human cost. Declines in job satisfaction, work–life balance and increasing work intensification contributed to the appearance of work-related stress as one of the key issues for workplace health and wellbeing. The 2008/09 recession further added to the concern of the working age population in terms of decreased perception of job security.

However, the preoccupation with ameliorating the malaise is set to change somewhat under current policy reforms regarding working age ill health and wellbeing. The perception that only 100 per cent fitness and work are compat-ible is set to be challenged, which marks the paradigmatic shift from negative to positive. No longer will the emphasis be on what people are unable to do. This applies to those in employment where discretionary alterations to duties can be applied, and also to those in unemployment and long-term incapacity. The message is consistent both in terms of working ill health reforms and welfare reforms: good health is good business and work always pays.

Yet, policy reform must not be seen as a panacea or a quick fix. Reform of this nature requires significant investment. Most importantly, there is a signifi-cant training need for line managers, general practitioners and human resource managers in dealing with the complexities of wellbeing in the working age population. Many of the beliefs and attitudes that people hold in relation to work-related wellbeing and ill health have been entrenched for generations. Therefore, considerable investment will be required in order to demonstrate the benefits of policy reform to key stakeholders and to ensure sustainability.

Bibliography

Ashkenas, R. (1999) 'Creating the Boundaryless Organization', *Business Horizons*, 42(5): 5–10.

Bell, D.N.F and Blanchflower, D.G. (2010) 'UK Unemployment in the Great Recession', *National Institute Economic Review*, 214(1): R3–R25.

Black, C. (2008) 'Working for a Healthier Tomorrow'. Available at http://www.dwp.gov.uk/docs/hwwb-working-for-a-healthier-tomorrow.pdf (accessed 16 February 2011).

Briner, R.B. and Reynolds, S. (1999) 'The Costs, Benefits and Limitations of Organizational Level Stress Interventions', *Journal of Organizational Behavior*, 20: 647–64.

Brockner, J., Grover, S., Reed, T. and DeWitt, R.L. (1992) 'Layoffs, Job Insecurity and Survivors' Work Effort: Evidence of an Inverted-U Relationship', *Academy of Management Journal*, 35: 413–25.

Clarke, A.E. (2011) 'Worker Well-Being in Booms and Busts', in P. Gregg and J. Wadsworth (eds), *The Labour Market in Winter: The State of Working Britain*. Oxford University Press: Oxford.

Coats, D. and Lekhi, R (2008) 'Good Jobs', cited in I. Brinkley, R. Fauth, M. Mahdon, and S. Theodoropoulou (2009), *Is Knowledge Work Better For Us? Knowledge Workers, Good Work and Wellbeing*. The Work Foundation. Available at http://www.theworkfoundation.com/assets/docs/publications/238_ke_wellbeing_final_final.pdf (accessed 16 February 2011).

Disney, R., Ratcliffe, A. and Smith, S. (2011) 'The Baby-Boomers at 50: Employment Prospects for Older Workers', in P. Gregg and J. Wadsworth (eds), *The Labour Market in Winter: The State of Working Britain*. Oxford: Oxford University Press.

Dolton, P. and Makepeace, G. (2011) 'Public and Private Sector Labour Markets', in P. Gregg and J. Wadsworth (eds), *The Labour Market in Winter: The State of Working Britain*. Oxford: Oxford University Press.

Dolton, P., Rosazza-Bondibene, C. and Wadsworth, J. (2011) 'The Regional Labour Market in the UK', in P. Gregg and J. Wadsworth (eds), *The Labour Market in Winter: The State of Working Britain*. Oxford: Oxford University Press.

Eason, K. (2002) 'People and Computers: Emerging Work Practice in the Information Age', in P. Warr (ed.), *Psychology at Work*. London: Penguin.

Faggio, G., Gregg, P. and Wadsworth, J. (2011) 'Job Tenure and Job Turnover', in P. Gregg and J. Wadsworth (eds), *The Labour Market in Winter: The State of Working Britain*. Oxford: Oxford University Press.

Feldman, D.C. (2007) 'Late Career and Retirement Issues', in H. Gunz and M. Peiperl (eds), *Handbook of Career Studies*. London: Sage.

Fineman, S. (2006) 'Accentuating the Positive?', *Academy of Management Review*, 31(2): 306–08.

Governmental Response to the Black Report (2008) 'Improving Health and Work: Changing Lives. The Government's Response to Dame Carol Black's Review of the Health of Britain's Working Age Population', Cmnd 7492. London: HMSO. Available at http://www.dwp.gov.uk/docs/hwwb-improving-health-and-work-changing-lives.pdf (accessed 16 February 2011).

Green, F. (2006) *Demanding Work: The Paradox of Job Quality in the Affluent Economy*. Princeton: Princeton University Press.

Green, F. (2011) 'Job Quality in Britain under the Labour Government', in P. Gregg and J. Wadsworth (eds), *The Labour Market in Winter: The State of Working Britain*. Oxford: Oxford University Press.

Gregg, P., Hansen, K. and Wadsworth, J. (1999) 'The Rise of the Workless Household', in P. Gregg and J. Wadsworth (eds), *The State of Working Britain*. Manchester: Manchester University Press.

Greller, M.M. and Stroh, L.K. (1995) 'Careers in Midlife and Beyond: A Fallow Field in Need of Sustenance', *Journal of Vocational Behavior*, 47: 232–47.

Guest, D.E. and Sturges, J. (2007) 'Living to Work – Working to Live', in H. Gunz, and M. Peiperl (eds), *Handbook of Career Studies*. London: Sage.

HSE (no date) "Health and Safety Executive Statistics 2009/10'. Available at http://www.hse.gov.uk/statistics/overall/hssh0910.pdf (accessed 27 February 2011).

HSE guidance online at http://www.hse.gov.uk/stress/furtheradvice/stressandmental health.htm (accessed 1 March 2011).

Jianli, W., Schmitz, N., Smailes, E., Sareen, J. and Patten, S. (2010) 'Work Characteristics, Depression and Health Related Presenteeism in a General Population Sample', *Journal of Occupational and Environmental Medicine*, 52(8): 836–42.

Johnson, S., Cooper, C., Cartwright, S., Donald, I., Taylor, P. and Millet, C. (2005) 'The Experience of Work Related Stress across Occupations', *Journal of Managerial Psychology*, 20(2): 178–87.

Kassenbaehmer, S.C. and Haisken-DeNew, J.P. (2009) 'You're Fired! The Causal Negative Effect of Entry Unemployment on Life Satisfaction', *Economic Journal*, 119(539): 448–62.

Kidd, J.M. (2002) 'Careers and Career Management', in P. Warr (eds), *Psychology at Work*. London: Penguin Books.

Knights, D. and McCabe, D. (1998) 'What Happens When The Phone Goes Wild? Staff, Stress and Spaces for Escape in a BPR Telephone Banking Work Regime', *Journal of Management Studies*, 35(2): 163–94.

Kuoppala, J., Lamminpaa, A. and Husman, P. (2008) 'Work Health Promotion, Job Well-Being and Sickness Absences. A Systematic Review and Meta-Analysis', *Journal of Occupational and Environmental Medicine*, 50(1): 1216–27.

Lin, X. and Leung, K. (2010) 'Differing Effects of Coping Strategies on Mental Health during Prolonged Unemployment: A Longitudinal Analysis', *Human Relations*, 63(5): 637–65.

Mills, P.R., Kessler, R.C., Cooper, J. and Sullivan, S. (2007) 'Impact of a Health Promotion Program on Employee Health Risks and Work Productivity' *American Journal of Health Promotion*, 22(1): 45–53.

O'Dowd, A. (2011) 'Job Losses are Likely as NHS Staff Reject Offer of National Pay Freeze', *British Medical Journal*, 342: d291.

ONS (Office of National Statistics) (2010) 'Workless Households'. Available at http://www.statistics.gov.uk/cci/nugget.asp?id=409 (accessed 25 February 2011).

ONS (Office of National Statistics) (2011a) 'Employment'. Available at http://www.statistics.gov.uk/cci/nugget.asp?id=12 (accessed 2 March 2011).

ONS (Office of National Statistics) (2011b) 'Older People in the Labour Market'. Available at http://www.statistics.gov.uk/cci/nugget.asp?id=2648 (accessed 2 March 2011).

Payne, J. (1987) 'Does Unemployment Run in Families? Some Findings from the General Household Survey', *Sociology*, 21(2): 199–214.

Payne, J. and Payne, C. (1994) 'Recession, Restructuring and the Fate of the Unemployed: Evidence in the Underclass Debate', *Sociology*, 28(1): 1–19.

Rank, M.R. and Cheng, L.C. (1995) 'Welfare Use across Generations: How Important are the Ties that Bind?', *Journal of Marriage and Family*, 57(3): 673–84.

Ranzijn, R., Carson, E., Winefield, A.H. and Price, D. (2006) 'On the Scrap Heap at 45: The Human Impact of Mature-Aged Unemployment', *Journal of Occupational and Organizational Psychology*, 79(3): 467–79.

Rick, J. and Briner, R.B. (2000) 'Psychosocial Risk Assessment: Problems and Prospects', *Occupational Medicine*, 50(5): 310–14.

Seligman, M.E.P. (1999) 'The President's Address', *American Psychologist*, 54: 250–63.

Sullivan, S. (1999) 'The Changing Nature of Careers: A Review and Research Agenda', *Journal of Management*, 25(3): 457–84.

Tucker, P., Brown, M., Dahlgren, A., Davies, G., Ebden, P., Folkard, S., Hutchings, H. and Akerstedt, T. (2010) 'The Impact of Junior Doctors' Work Time Arrangements on their Fatigue and Wellbeing', *Scandinavian Journal of Work Environmental Health*, 36(6): 458–65.

Waddell, G. and Burton, K.A. (2006) 'Is Work Good for your Health and Well-Being?', A Review commissioned by DWP. London: TSO.

Waterhouse, J.M., Folkard, S. and Minors, D.S. (1992) 'Shiftwork, Health and Safety: An Overview of the Scientific Literature 1978–1990'. London: HMSO.

Wester, G.. and Wolff, J. (2010) 'The Social Gradient in Health: How Fair Retirement could Make a Difference', *Public Health Ethics*, 3(3): 272–81.

Winkleman, R. (2008) 'Unemployment, Social Capital and Subjective Wellbeing', *Journal of Happiness Studies*, 10(4): 421–30.

Working Futures 2007–2017 (no date) Available at http://www.ukces.org.uk/upload/pdf/15236%209%20UKCES%20Executive%20Summary%202.%20Working%20Futures_2.pdf.

Workplace Employee Relations Survey (2004) Available at http://www.berr.gov.uk/files/file11423.pdf (accessed 16 February 2011).

Wellbeing and Community Action

8

Dafydd Thomas

The aim of this chapter is to explore links between community development and community wellbeing. It explores what community development, community engagement and community wellbeing mean, and how it is possible to combine them. It also looks at different community engagement techniques that would promote greater wellbeing, and concludes by considering what needs to happen at local and national government to make these wellbeing interventions happen as a matter of routine, rather than as exceptional instances of good practice.

Engaging and developing communities

I would argue that the public sector sees its role mainly in terms of providing services for its clients. This provider–client perspective gives rise to a culture of 'needs,' to be met by the expert interventions of 'professionals'. But such expert intervention is costly, expends increasingly limited financial resources and is, thus, ultimately financially unsustainable.

In contrast, there is a movement of community development, engagement and empowerment workers that feels that connecting with users requires something much deeper than merely satisfying the needs of consumers of a service. Indeed, this movement would feel that community involvement should be recognized as being 'a fundamental civil right', as described by Burton (2004: 193–8).

What is community development?

According to the Community Development Foundation and the New Economics Foundation (2010: 3) 'Community Development is a way of working with local communities, to achieve change within communities to problems that they themselves identify. It is a collective process, not a one off intervention, co-produced with, not for, communities.'

In other words, community development provides individuals and groups of people with the skills to engage in processes that develop a collective vision of benefits for that community. Community engagement is the final outcome, where agencies have an ongoing, dynamic, mutually beneficial relationship with a community or an individual.

These descriptions of community development illustrate a dynamic process with a range of processes and interventions. This, in turn, has resulted in a range of interpretations by different organizations of who controls what. And here lies a problem for all the participants in a community engagement scenario.

The well-documented ladder of engagement by Arnstein (1969: 216–24) provides a model to explain the different levels of citizen involvement and participation with another, service providing, organization (Figure 8.1). Various and increasingly complex theories of participation have been used to further characterize this ladder or spectrum of participation and engagement. At one end of the scale are the 'clients' responding to 'service provider' manipulation or cynical misinformation. At the other end of the scale, Bovaird and Downe (no date) describe a scenario where all the stakeholders are taking part in local, bottom up, strategic decision-making processes.

For the purpose of this chapter, I would like to emphasize the point that organizations can choose different levels of engagement with their client group

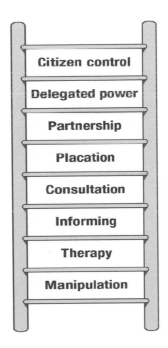

Figure 8.1   Arnstein's ladder of citizen participation

Source: Arnstein (1969), reproduced with the permission of Taylor & Francis.

or local population – which could fit somewhere on the Arnstein model or one of its derivatives.

Community development practitioners would argue that communities are actually a resource in themselves. Whether these communities represent a specific geographic area or special interest, they contain a wealth of drive, energy, knowledge and imagination that could be combined with the financial resources historically available only to the public sector. Often, key individuals are needed to oil the wheels in this process and this role is often undertaken by a community development officer.

According to the Community Development Foundation and the New Economics Foundation (2010: 3), the role of the community development worker is to 'enable, facilitate and build capacity for a community to address its own needs'. Coopers and Lybrand (1999) describe the role of the community development worker as being to 'empower [individuals] to change things by developing their own skills, knowledge and experience, and also by working in partnerships with other groups and with statutory agencies'.

Coopers and Lybrand further define community development as:

> strengthening and bringing about change in communities. It consists of a set of methods which can broaden vision and capacity for social change and approaches including consultation, advocacy and relationships with local groups. It is a way of working, informed by certain principles which seek to encourage communities ... to tackle for themselves the problems which they face and identify to be important.

With such a range of techniques available to the community development worker and the different interpretations of engagement characterized by Arnstein and others, it is not surprising that the prevailing public sector view of providing an expert service to their 'clients' still persists. It is a complicated and complex area of work which often puts decision-makers off. But changes are happening. A key recommendation from Marmot *et al.* (2010: 15) was for effective local delivery to have 'effective participatory decision-making at a local level'. The review goes on to say, 'This can only happen by empowering individuals and local communities.'

For the rest of this chapter, I will try to provide a basic rule of thumb for the kind of community development practices or interventions that I believe increase the wellbeing of the communities involved. I will also provide some evidence of why I believe these practices can improve community wellbeing.

Community wellbeing: subjective and objective wellbeing

When thinking about wellbeing in the context of communities – and that of community development and engagement, in particular – I find the definition used by Felce and Perry (1995: 51–74) most useful. They describe two dimensions to wellbeing – the objective and subjective:

- objective wellbeing means the social and material attributes that contribute or detract from an individual or community's wellbeing. These include wealth, provision of health care or education, infrastructure and so on;
- subjective wellbeing is related to an individual's assessment of their own circumstances: what they think and feel. It is an area that has produced a great deal of activity amongst psychologists and economists.

(These aspects of wellbeing are described in greater detail in Chapter 2.)

Using these definitions, it is easy to imagine a theoretical, mutually beneficial, circumstance promoting wellbeing where both service provider and the local community are recognized as, at the very least, equal partners in the decision-making process. For example, a situation where individuals within the community are able to contribute their own energy and ideas to decisions and subsequent actions that enhance a local agency's activities within their community can only benefit both parties. According to Felce and Perry's definition, the subjective wellbeing of these individuals will improve, because they are given the opportunity to articulate openly what they think and feel about a decision, how it impacts on their lives, affects their aspirations and whether it gives them a role in delivering the proposed changes. Equally, their objective wellbeing would improve, as the service would be better suited to address their social, material and economic needs because it is better informed and owned by members of that community.

Evidence exists that corroborates this theoretical win–win situation. The New Economics Foundation (2004: 2) estimates that 40 per cent of an individual's wellbeing is dependent on their outlook and activities, where individuals 'have the most opportunity to make a difference to wellbeing'. They conclude that community involvement is also a very important contributing factor to wellbeing.

The New Economics Foundation was commissioned to develop a set of evidence-based actions that would help improve personal wellbeing as part of the UK Government's Foresight programme's 2008 Mental Capital and Wellbeing Project. They came up with *Five Ways to Wellbeing* (2008) (see Chapter 2), which reflected the key findings from the evidence base in the form of five actions that could improve personal wellbeing. Two of those key actions demonstrate the win–win benefits available to community wellbeing, if the public sector chooses to let local citizens have greater control in the decision-making process and so support the co-designing of the final outcome. These are:

- *Connect* with the people around you … in your local community. Think of these as the cornerstones of your life and invest time in developing them. Building these connections will support and enrich you every day; and
- *Give* Do something nice for a friend, or a stranger. Volunteer your time. Join a community group. Look out, as well as in. Seeing yourself, and your happiness, linked to the wider community can be incredibly rewarding and will create connections with the people around you.

Both individual and community 'connecting' and 'giving' could be added to the resources available to support local action and inform local decisions.

Adopting Felce and Perry's framework, there would also be a wellbeing dividend at the subjective and objective levels in a local community/public sector service delivery partnership.

Individual capabilities

Another approach is to consider wellbeing in the context of an individual's ability to cope. If an individual is unable to cope, their wellbeing suffers. But what determines an individual's ability to cope?

Hall and Taylor (2009: 83) describe an individual's ability to cope as depending on how the individual responds to the 'life challenges' they face. It is these life challenges that impact upon an individual's health and wellbeing through a daily process of wear and tear. Each individual response it based upon two factors:

- a person's personality, emotional resilience, reflective consciousness and self-esteem; and
- the ability that person has to elicit cooperation from others.

So, if your life is full of challenges but you do not have the capabilities to deal with them, higher levels of stress and anxiety are likely, leading to poorer levels of physical and mental health that will ultimately impact upon your personal wellbeing and, most probably, the wellbeing of those around you. According to Hall and Taylor, these challenges are influenced by social and economic factors, which can make it harder for an individual to cope with increasingly difficult circumstances.

Communities are more than collections of individuals. But if those individuals cannot cooperate or work together because they are less practised in the art, then I believe that a community can descend into a collection of self-interested individuals, with a negative impact on community wellbeing as a result.

In order to avoid that scenario, it is possible to imagine a community worker being able to improve an individual's own capabilities and wellbeing directly, and the community wellbeing indirectly, by working within a community. If people are given the tools and capacity to help them contribute to cooperative decisions within their community, this kind of intervention has the potential to make a considerable impact.

Evidence from research would indicate that this is the case:

- Mutual cooperation is associated with enhanced neuronal response in the reward areas of the brain, which indicates that social cooperation is intrinsically rewarding, according to Rilling *et al.* (in New Economics Foundation, 2008: 10).
- Greenfield and Marks (in New Economics Foundation, 2008: 10) found that, for older people, volunteering is associated with more positive affect and more meaning in life.
- Wellbeing is described by the New Economics Foundation (2008: 1) as having two main elements: 'feeling good and functioning well'. Feelings of

happiness, contentment, enjoyment, curiosity and engagement are characteristic of someone who has a positive experience of their life. Equally
important for wellbeing is day-to-day functioning. Experiencing positive
relationships, having some control over one's life and having a sense of
purpose are all important attributes of wellbeing.

So, individuals with low self-esteem, poor reflective skills and low emotional
resilience could be supported by a community development worker in some
guise, in order to improve their own wellbeing and that of the community at
large. This fits in well with Coopers and Lybrand's (1999) definition of a community development worker mentioned earlier as someone who empowers individuals to change things by developing their own skills, knowledge and experience.

The New Economic Foundation (2004: 16) concurs. 'Research shows
clearly that we derive wellbeing from engaging with one another in meaningful projects ... the personal development aspect of wellbeing is likely to be
linked with engaging actively with life and our communities.'

In considering the 'ideal empowering authority', Local Government
Improvement and Development (2010: 2) supports community engagement
and community empowerment because they deliver:

- resilient communities with strong social networks and active citizens
  taking responsibility for their own wellbeing;
- vibrant democracy; and
- better services.

To conclude, there are many different ways of working with a geographic or
special interest community. Some ways of working have the potential to
improve individual and collective wellbeing either through the means of
engagement, through the type of service provided as a result of that engagement
process, or by building the capabilities of individuals within a specific community as a specific action of the engagement process. When there are always pressures on the public purse, an agency or public sector body must ask itself:

- In which situations should an intervention of some type occur?
- What techniques are available that will increase citizen control, share
  resources and generate inclusive decisions that deliver what is needed for
  all concerned, but in a way that benefits the collective wellbeing of the
  communities and organizations involved?

The next section will attempt to answer those questions.

Community engagement as a wellbeing intervention

In order to improve community wellbeing, from the start, public sector organizations need to take the following factors into account when developing a
service in partnership with their target community:

- designing services with wellbeing in mind;
- how to measure their impact;
- where to put their effort; and
- what community engagement techniques can be used to maximize community wellbeing and deliver well-designed and well-delivered services that benefit the public and its partners.

Designing services with wellbeing in mind

We have seen in the previous section the wellbeing benefits from proper community engagement and involvement. We have also discussed the need to build the capabilities within communities so that they can make a useful contribution to the decisions that affect and shape them. Finally, evidence demonstrates that services tailored to the needs of their communities contribute to improvements in that community's objective wellbeing.

But why go to such an effort?

As described in Chapters 2 and 4, for local authorities, Section 2(1) of the Local Government Act 2000 places a legal duty on them to promote the economic, social and environmental wellbeing of their areas. Part 1 of the same act, provides the means to do so through the community strategy process, using the discretionary wellbeing power.

The Local Government Act 2000 was part of a local authority reform process, linked to a wider reform of public services agenda of the UK government at that time. According to the Department for Communities and Local Government (1999), the aim of the reform was to provide services to the public that were:

- better co-ordinated;
- responsive to the needs and concerns of local communities;
- delivered in ways that suit the people who depended on them; and
- took account of the needs of future generations.

(For further detail on the role and responsibilities of local government for wellbeing, see Chapter 4.)

Apart from the legal duty enshrined in the Local Government Act, there is compelling evidence for wanting better engagement between communities and the public services. For instance, Professor John Mc Knight (2010) believes that public sector organizations need to work more closely with local communities because they have reached the limits of their effectiveness working alone. Ng and Ho (2006: 1) feel that public policy needs to enhance the happiness or welfare of the people both now and in the future, otherwise 'if public policy reduces or is neutral with regard to happiness, why go through the trouble of designing and implementing all kinds of policies?' Hall and Taylor (2009: 83) argue that public policies affect collective wellbeing through their impact on the structure of social relations. They believe that these social relations are resources on which individuals draw to advance their own welfare. In short, Hall and Taylor see public policymaking as a process of social resource creation, and social resources as central to population health and wellbeing.

So, whether for reasons of better service delivery, or as part of an overt attempt to improve the public's subjective and objective wellbeing, public services should be designed in cooperation with their target audience – with improving wellbeing as the over-riding aim. When the public sector openly discusses how to improve wellbeing with its stakeholders, the New Economics Foundation (2009: 14) has found that the concept resonates with what people care about. Its broad appeal and understanding also helps inform choices that face communities about decisions that impact upon overall community wellbeing. The New Economics Foundation sees measuring wellbeing as a key step in engaging that wide audience of stakeholders.

Case study: the *Exploring Sustainable Wellbeing Toolkit*

In order to do this, the Wellbeing Wales Network has developed the Exploring Sustainable Wellbeing Toolkit that makes sustainable wellbeing a central aim in the planning and delivery of a project or service (for further details, visit www.wellbeingwales.org).

The *Exploring Sustainable Wellbeing Toolkit* was designed to help organizations consider sustainable wellbeing in a practical, interactive and thought provoking way. It is a conversation-based process that works best during the development phase of an idea, project or programme of work. The six-stage process helps organizations think about wellbeing in the context of their own

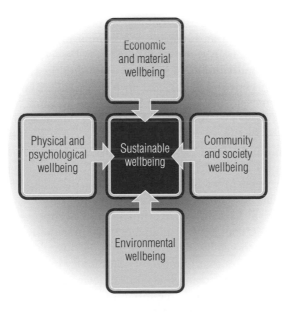

Figure 8.2   Model used in the *Exploring Sustainable Wellbeing Toolkit*

work; assess the current wellbeing impact of what is planned; think about alternatives; prioritize how to do things differently before fleshing out those plans and evaluating their impact.

The Toolkit uses a holistic model of wellbeing (see Figure 8.2), which provides the basis for wide-ranging discussion when participants are using the process. In developing the Toolkit, participants were able to articulate what wellbeing meant to them personally and in the context of what they were trying to achieve. Going through the process, participants were able to see what wellbeing meant in the practical delivery of their project or plan. The Toolkit's engaging and practical nature means that it makes the delivery of wellbeing something that everyone can relate to and not just an area for policy and academic analysis.

Measuring subjective wellbeing within communities

It goes without saying that, if the outcome of public policy delivery is to improve wellbeing, some measure of the impacts of a particular policy would help assess its usefulness to communities and society at large. Measuring the subjective wellbeing of local communities would be a very useful tool in assessing effective policy delivery and should be at the heart of the decision-making process.

The focus of this chapter has been to look at the wider wellbeing benefits possible as part of a public service intervention that seeks to engage and encourage community participation in the decision-making process. As we have seen, any such intervention can either promote wellbeing or ill-being, which has inevitable consequences. The question is where to put the effort.

It would seem reasonable and humane to provide the most disadvantaged members of society with an intensive community development type of inter-vention that would benefit those communities collectively in terms of service co-design, but also individually in terms of providing the skills to deal with the life challenges that Hall and Taylor (2009: 83) describe. But it is not just about focusing on the most deprived communities. For instance, the more 'profes-sional' members of society, higher up the social gradient, also have restrictions on their ability to engage in decisions that have considerable effect on them and their communities. The Canadian Index of Wellbeing (2010) describes the 'Time Crunch' as a phenomenon where people's time for anything other than work is being eroded by technologies that erase the boundaries between the workplace and home. Put another way, Wheatley (in 'The New Economics Foundation', Welsh Assembly Government and Wellbeing Wales Network, 2008) found that 72 per cent of managers say that their long hours restrict their opportunities to get involved in community life. Public sector decision-makers need to be aware that one size of community involvement aimed at the more deprived and those lacking life capabilities will not fit all circumstances.

Other issues – such as improvement in child care, equal pay for women and the lack of opportunity for low-income families – play their part in restricting people's involvement in the decisions that affect their community. These factors need to be considered when deciding which technique should be used to engage with the community of interest, thereby improving local wellbeing.

The Marmot Review's promotion of 'proportionate universalism' would seem to be an appropriate response, where interventions occur on 'a scale and intensity that is proportionate to the level of disadvantage' (Marmot, 2010). Marmot is concerned with the health inequalities that exist within our society, yet the principle is equally applicable to inequalities in wellbeing. Using a measure of subjective wellbeing across our society would be appropriate to determine which areas are disadvantaged and deserving of a higher intensity wellbeing intervention. At the higher end of the economic scale where levels of wellbeing are unknown, different, potentially less intense types of intervention would be required by the public sector in its decision-making process.

How the public sector should work to improve long-term wellbeing

As the public sector could never have all the resources it would like, any intervention by that sector – or any other agency, for that matter – needs to be effective to ensure maximum cost effectiveness. An additional challenge is to make such interventions long-lasting and, ultimately, self-sustaining. So, how can the public sector and other agencies change from doing things to their communities to doing things with the communities and promoting greater wellbeing as an intentional consequence?

Using Arnstein's ladder of citizen participation (1969), I believe that the greater level of citizen control or involvement wherever possible, when dealing with the public sector, the greater the levels of subjective wellbeing accrued by the community (see Figure 8.3). Or, in other words, rather than the public sector being a producer of a service with the local community being a distinct

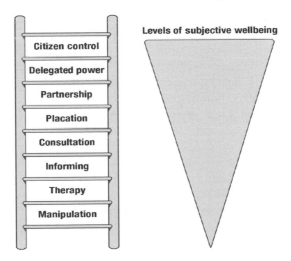

Figure 8.3   The ladder of citizen participation and increasing subjective wellbeing

Source: Arnstein (1969), reproduced with the permission of Taylor & Francis.

consumer, those lines and definitions need to become less distinct. The local community can be both a producer and consumer of a service, with the public sector or other agency's role being one to facilitate that change or individual involvement. In addition, I believe that citizen control ultimately delivers services that are better suited to their needs, so improving objective wellbeing as a result.

Based on my assessment of some of the current community development techniques being practised in the UK, I have produced the following list as a practical guide as to what wellbeing promoting community engagement and collaboration looks like. These techniques should be used by an organization at the start of the decision-making process, not bolted on at the end. That way, the community would be an equal partner and provider of rich resources to support the agency's activity with the community:

- *Time banking*: where everyone's contribution is valued equally. This is based on the principles that everyone has something worthwhile to contribute and that for each hour a person contributes they earn an hour's credit. This credit can then be used to access services and support offered by other time bank participants, which then becomes a basis for exchange of goods or services. Time banks build up a sense of community by using time as a medium of exchange.
- *Co-production*: where users and providers pool different kinds of knowledge and skills to produce a service that meets everyone's needs. According to the New Economic Foundation's Green Well Fair (2009: 13), the resources used are 'available in abundance within our local communities – priceless resources such as time, wisdom, experience, energy, knowledge and skills'. They go on to say that co-production can 'transform people's relationships with their own wellbeing because it enables them to feel valued and to have more control over what happens'.
- *Asset-based community development* (www.abcdinstitute.org): challenges the view that communities are broken or in need. When communities are described as being in need, this develops a dependency culture within that community where things need to be fixed by outside interventions. Asset-based community development considers a community as having assets that are the primary building blocks of sustainable community development. There are five kinds of assets within a community that can be drawn upon to build stronger, more sustainable communities for the future:
  o *talents and skills of people* – that can be nurtured and developed;
  o *associations and networks of people* – in which the talents of individuals can be magnified;
  o *institutions and professional entities*;
  o *physical assets such as land or property*; and
  o *local economic assets such as local business* – which can support exchanges (often non-monetary).
- *Cooperatives or mutual aid organizations*: According to the Wales Cooperative Centre (www.walescoop.com), a cooperative is quite simply a business that is owned and controlled by its members. The formal definition from the International Co-operative Alliance is 'An autonomous association

of persons united voluntarily to meet their common economic, social, and cultural needs and aspirations through a jointly-owned and democratically-controlled enterprise.' These types of organizations are used by social landlords or in providing food within local communities.

Implications for government policy: flip the paradigm

As discussed at the start of this chapter, the prevailing public sector view is that they provide services to needy client communities, and that without the expert intervention of paid officers, the client community members would flounder. Historically, community groups cannot access the financial resources available to the public sector, yet they contain a wealth of energy, ideas and potential that remains untapped. Looking at co-production as an example, the New Economics Foundation (2009: 13) sees priceless resources such as time, wisdom, experience, energy, knowledge and skills that, on the whole, remain untapped and unused. The paradigm of needy communities needs to be turned on its head. For example, the Community Development Foundation and the New Economics Foundation (2010: 5) found that, for each £1 invested in community development activities, £2.16 of social and economic value is created. They have also found that, for every £1 that a local authority invests in a community development worker, £6 of value is contributed by community members in volunteering time.

Local Government Improvement and Development (2010: 47) sees the role of local government as being 'about providing the infrastructure support to enable individuals and communities to develop an environment that promotes their wellbeing'. They feel that, to do this effectively, local councils need to:

- 'be more outward looking, to allow people's experience of local life to be a key driver of activity.' Is this a measure of subjective wellbeing by another name?;
- remember that their role extends beyond that of service provider. They emphasize the role of community engagement, including 'listening to citizen's views about local priorities' and 'harnessing people's knowledge, skills and enthusiasm to co-create solutions that bring benefits to all';
- recognize the value the resources of individuals, families and social networks that communities bring to the table and which sustain society;
- see their role as 'facilitating solutions', which could be to include appropriate community engagement wellbeing interventions targeted on communities according to their subjective wellbeing score;
- 'Think less about their local population as passive recipients of services and more about them as agents of change.'

The document goes even further, to state that all levels of government could promote wellbeing by 'fostering an asset-based approach; encouraging social relationships between families, communities and citizens and enhancing local action'.

So, the message is that communities have resources and that the way the public sector fosters these is key to shifting from a community with needs to one capable of helping to transform its own future.

Support individuals and their communities appropriately

The role of community participation and engagement in public decision-making processes has received increasing interest, witness references made to this approach in the Welsh Assembly Government's 'Making the Connections' policy (2005); the subsequent 'Beyond Boundaries: Citizen-Centred Local Services for Wales' action plan (2006) and the 'Communities First Programme'. More recent interests include the Conservative Party's call for a Big Society (2010) and the Marmot Review on Health Inequalities (Marmot, 2010).

As mentioned, there are various ways in which individuals within a community are hampered from taking an active part within their communities and contributing to its overall wellbeing. As a result, public sector partners need to use a range of means to engage with these individuals – either through direct support, improving individual skills to cooperate, or by being more creative in how the sector communicates with its target audience. Often, the direct intervention of a community development worker ensures that the appropriate means of interaction is developed between partners.

Hothi *et al.* (2010: 5), on behalf of the Young Foundation, found through its Wellbeing Project that the most powerful forms of empowerment were 'those that aimed to maximize the capabilities of the local people, rather than simply devolving decisions from one group to another'. As a result, wellbeing increased.

Hothi *et al.*'s (2010: 7–10) analysis particularly emphasizes the value of:

- providing greater opportunities for residents to influence decisions affecting their neighbourhoods;
- facilitating regular contact between neighbours; and
- helping residents gain the confidence they need to exercise control over local circumstances.

Make greater use of the wellbeing power

Section 2(1) of the Local Government Act 2000 provides local authorities with a discretionary power to do anything that they consider is likely to achieve the promotion or improvement of the economic, social and environmental wellbeing of their areas.

According to a review by the Department for Communities and Local Government in a recent review on the use of this wellbeing power (2008: 1), its use 'remained limited over the life of the evaluation'. It went on to say that 'policy makers needed to be more explicit in their usage and in identifying opportunities for the use of the power in their policy proposals'. Using the wellbeing power to resource the measurement of subjective wellbeing would be a good start, followed by the establishment of a legally binding cooperative or time bank that responded to the community's identified requirements. The report concluded that:

the many and varied ways in which awareness and understanding of the wellbeing power translate into use and are affected by a range of factors including:

- the capacity and capability of the local authority
- the strength of local partnership relationships and
- the nature of interactions between the centre and the locality.

So, once again, the type and strength of relationship between an authority and its communities is key to using the power. It would also appear that there is a capacity issue within local government to relinquish the power they hold and develop the capability to work with and engage their local communities.

Complete commitment

The Department for Communities and Local Government's review (2008: 6) concludes that there is a 'need for policy makers to attend to implementation at the "top" as well as "bottom", and reinforce the importance of communication, clarity and consistency in dealings between the centre and localities throughout the implementation process'. So, the final pieces of this jigsaw puzzle are for the public service to realize its impact on promoting community wellbeing; use a wellbeing promoting community engagement technique; and, most importantly, take a whole organization approach to the issue. This is too great an opportunity to be relegated to the usual suspects – namely, the more progressive members of a local authority, health board or NHS trust.

Conclusion

The thrust of this chapter has been to illustrate that, by using community development and engagement techniques, it is possible to improve the wellbeing of our communities. Such an approach promotes further engagement and ties together different agendas and policy areas. Investing in the capabilities of individuals and supporting the involvement of communities as equal partners in the delivery of a particular service or activity will both improve the service and increase the cohesion of that community. Finally, such an approach has an extremely healthy financial return.

There has been a great deal of discussion recently about empowerment and engagement in relation to public sector delivery. But is this mere civic hype? Are those in power willing to relinquish power and lose control of their grand vision? Decision-makers must realize that they have a different role to play in today's society, and that it is time to grasp the engagement nettle. Otherwise, we will continue to pour resources into communities with little hope of improving anyone's wellbeing.

Bibliography

Arnstein, S. (1969) 'A Ladder of Citizen Participation', *Journal of the American Institute of Planners*, 35: 216–24.

Bovaird, T. and Downe, J. (no date) 'Innovation in Public Engagement and Co-production of services, Meta-Evaluation of the Local Government Modernisation Agenda – White Paper Policy Paper'. Available at www.cardiff.ac.uk/carbs/research/groups/clrgr/policypaper.pdf.

Burton, P. (2004) 'Power to the People? How to Judge Public Participation', *Local Economy*, 19(3): 193–8.

Canadian Index of Wellbeing (June 2010) 'Caught in the Time Crunch: Time Use Leisure and Culture in Canada'.

Community Development Foundation and the New Economics Foundation (2010) 'Catalysts for Community Action and Investment: A Social Return on Investment Analysis of Community Development Work, based on a Common Outcomes Framework, October.

Coopers and Lybrand (1999) 'Department of Health and Social Services', Baseline Study of Community Development approaches to Health and Social Wellbeing. Coopers and Lybrand.

Department for Communities and Local Government (1999) 'Preparing Community Strategies: Government Guidance to Local Authorities', 8 December.

Department for Communities and Local Government (2008) 'Practical Use of the Wellbeing Power', 17 November.

Felce, D. and Perry, J. (1995) 'Quality of Life: Its Definition and Measurement', *Research Developmental Disabilities*, 16(1): 51–74.

Greenfield, E.A. and Marks, N.F. (2004) 'Formal Volunteering as a Protective Factor for Older Adults' Psychological Well-Being', *Journals of Gerontology, Series B: Psychological Sciences and Social Sciences*, 59B: 258–64. Hall, P. and Taylor, R. (2009) 'Health Social Relations and Public Policy Successful Stories: How Institutions and Culture affect Health', Cambridge University: 83.

Holt-Lunstad, J., Smith, T.B. and Layton, J.B. (2010)' Social Relationships and Mortality Risk: A Meta-analytic Review', *PLoS Medicine*, 7(7). Available at e1000316. doi:10.1371/journal.pmed.1000316.

Hothi, M., with Bacon, N., Brophy, M. and Mulgan, G. (2008) *Neighbourliness + Empowerment = Wellbeing: Is there a Formula for Happy Communities*. London: Young Foundation on behalf of the Wellbeing Project.

Local Government Improvement and Development (LGID) (2010) *The Ideal Empowering Authority: An Illustrated Framework*. London: Local Government Improvement and Development.

Local Government Improvement and Development (LGID) and the National Mental Health Development Unit (NMHDU) Written by the New Economics Foundation Local Government Improvement and Development (2010) 'The Role of Local Government in Promoting Wellbeing', November.

Marmot, M. *et al.* (2010) 'Fair Society, Healthy Lives: The Marmot Review, Strategic Review of Health Inequalities post-2010'. Available at http://www.marmotreview.org.

McKnight, Prof. John (2010) of the Asset Based Community Development Institute in the School of Education and Social Policy in North Western University, Illinois stated in UKPHA's Public Health Forum, March.

New Economics Foundation (2004) 'A Wellbeing Manifesto for a Flourishing Society'. New Economics Foundation.

New Economics Foundation (2008) 'Five Ways to Wellbeing', October. New Economics Foundation.

New Economics Foundation (2009a) 'Green Well Fair – Three Economies for Social Justice', February. New Economics Foundation.

New Economics Foundation (2009b) 'National Accounts of Wellbeing: Bringing Real Wealth onto the Balance Sheet', January. New Economics Foundation.

Ng, Y.-K. and Ho, L.S. (2006) 'Introduction: Happiness as the Only Ultimate Objective of Public Policy', in Y.-K. Ng and Ho, L.S., *Happiness and Public Policy: Theory, Case Studies and Implications*. New York: Palgrave Macmillan: 1–16.

Rilling, J., Glenn, A., Jairam, M., Pagnoni, G., Goldsmith, D., Elfenbein, H. and Lilienfeld, S. (2007) 'Neural Correlates of Social Cooperation and Non-Cooperation as a Function of Psychopathy', *Biological Psychiatry*, 61(11): 1260–71.

Wheatley, R. (2000) *Taking the Strain: A Survey of Managers and Workplace Stress*. London: Institute of Management.

Partnership Working: The Lynchpin of Wellbeing

9

Mike Ponton and Marie John

This chapter reviews our current state of understanding of collaboration in the form of partnerships, alliances and networks. Adopting a theoretical perspective informed by experience drawn from recent action research carried out by the Welsh Institute of Health and Social Care (WIHSC) that focused on improving multi-agency collaboration in Wales, it first considers the contexts and conditions under which collaborative activity can flourish, and then goes on to investigate how collaboration is sustained.

Introduction

Organizations can do things that no individual can do by themselves. The truth of this statement is demonstrated throughout history. From the building of Stonehenge to the construction of the Eiffel Tower, people have worked together to achieve collective results beyond their personal limitations. Groups of organizations can do things that no organization can do by itself. But the history of human collaboration is decidedly chequered. Inter-governmental action on poverty and climate control has been obstructed by self-interest. Other difficult problems that have yet to be solved by multi-sectoral actions include drug and alcohol abuse. Solving these problems – or even agreeing that they exist – has moved centre-stage in international and national government policy. The question naturally arises: Do we have theories or practical knowledge about collaboration that can be successfully applied in a variety of contexts?

The idea of partnership working in the field of health is not new. The 1977 World Health Assembly called for Health for All by the year 2000 and proposed, in the Alma-Ata Declaration of 1978, that a primary care led

movement with partnership at its heart would be the strategy for the achievement of this objective. At the core of this movement was the drive to work for
a more equal world and the improvement of the health status of the world's
poorest nations. Inter-sectoral collaboration – in other words, a partnership
between all sectors – was central to the success of the strategy.

The World Health Organization's Ottawa Charter (WHO, 1986) describes
health promotion as the process of enabling people to increase control over,
and to improve, their health. To reach a state of complete physical, mental and
social wellbeing, an individual or group must be able to:

- identify and to realize aspirations;
- satisfy needs; and
- change, or cope with, the environment.

Health is seen as a resource for everyday life, not the objective of living. Health
is a positive concept emphasizing social and personal resources, as well as
physical capacities. Therefore, health promotion is not just the responsibility
of the health sector; it goes beyond healthy lifestyles to wellbeing. The Charter
proposed five areas for priority action in promoting health, and these give a
framework for considering the promotion of wellbeing:

- building healthy public policy;
- creating supportive environments;
- strengthening community actions;
- developing personal skills; and
- reorienting health services.

In terms of statutory services in the UK, partnership working in the field of
health and social care has been actively promoted as a policy issue since 1974,
when the public health and community health care functions of local authorities were transferred to the NHS. In the field of public health, however, this
is a much more recent development in the wake of the 'Health for All' (1978)
initiative and the Black Report (1980). The growing understanding of the role
of the wider determinants of health, particularly since the 1990s, has resulted
in increasing emphasis on 'joined up' (i.e. partnership) working. Various
provisions to encourage joint working, including the potentially very important provision of pooled budgets, were made in the 1999 Health Act. These
incorporated a range of initiatives including health action zones, health
improvement programmes and the placing of a specific duty on primary care
trusts to promote partnership working. This resulted in greater interaction
between the NHS, local authorities and the voluntary sector in the cause of
improving health and wellbeing. This interaction was facilitated by the Local
Government Act 2000, which gave local authorities the power to promote
social, economic and environmental wellbeing. These developments met with
variable success; among the factors that have been identified as determining
their effectiveness are the extent to which partner organizations have historically worked together; the level of trust between the partners; co-terminosity

of boundaries across organizations; having shared targets, incentives and performance assessment systems; and arrangements relating to shared resources.

Co-terminosity has been an issue in the UK at least since 1974 and continues to be one that is seen as an important determinant of effective collaboration. It is particularly an issue in England, where the continued existence of two-tier local government causes major problems. In Wales and Scotland, co-terminosity between the major public sector players was achieved several years ago. Co-terminosity is less relevant to collaboration between the public and voluntary sectors, which has proved much more difficult to achieve because of, among other factors, the pluralist nature of the sector and the understandable resistance of individual voluntary organizations to adopting a common agenda.

Partnership in the public sector

In the National Leadership and Innovation Agency for Healthcare's publication, 'Working in Collaboration: Learning from Theory and Practice' (2007), Williams and Sullivan report that, in the UK, the need for coordination in government stems, in part:

- from the fragmentation of public services, and the creation of multiple agencies with unclear and differing forms of accountability;
- from the fact that government, in general, has tended to intervene in more aspects of society and the economy;
- from the continuing fiscal problems, which place a premium on the need to secure economic efficiency and best use of resources;
- as a result of decentralization and devolution, which make problems of coordination and policy coherence between different tiers of governance highly problematic; and
- as a consequence of the increasing globalization of policy issues.

There have been sporadic attempts over successive decades to secure better coordination in government and public policy but, in recent times, there has been a proliferation of activity across a wide policy front, including crime and community safety, children and young people, the environment, health, housing, education and transport. Dowling *et al.* (2004) state: 'it is difficult to find a contemporary policy document or set of good practice guidelines that does not have collaboration as the central strategy for the delivery of welfare'. McMurray (2007) suggests that government policy in the UK, while extolling the virtues of a partnership approach, is guilty of undermining it through perpetual organizational reforms that destroy often delicate communication channels, decision processes and inter-organizational relationships. In addition, the nature of many reforms based on contestability, markets and contracts, together with their prescriptive form, means that 'actors at all levels are required to divert attention from long-term processes, such as boundary spanning activities, as they are directed or incentivised by central government to deal with that which is politically urgent or organisationally new' (McMurray, 2007: 79).

Williams and Sullivan (2007) also tell us that the emphasis on partnership working has been precipitated by a range of policy instruments based on forms of collaboration and partnership that are cross-sectoral in nature, involve all major policy areas, are applicable at all levels of governance, and are appropriate at different stages of the policy process.

Partnership – both across social care and health, and also with service users – has been a key theme of the modernization agenda. Despite a relatively underdeveloped evidence base, the establishment of health and social care partnerships has featured strongly in recent policy and legislative initiatives. Also, the emphasis on working in partnership with users and carers to achieve individual choice and to maximize independence has become ever more important. This, and the growing understanding of the role of the wider determinants of health and wellbeing, particularly since the 1990s, has resulted in increasing emphasis on 'joined up' partnership working, and is now a central part of public health policy across the UK.

The Deputy Prime Minister's Strategic Partnering Taskforce Guide (2006) pointed out that most of local government spending involves a choice. This choice might mean procuring from suppliers of goods, works and services; and it might mean entering into a partnership with the private sector. However, increasingly as a means to achieve best value, the choice may be a public/public partnership. Providing services to communities requires all authorities to question whether they should deliver these services themselves or with others – the so-called 'make or buy' decision. In the 1990s, for many councils, especially those providing the full range of local government services, the likely answer was 'the 'make' option (i.e. let's do it in-house), but sometimes 'the buy' option (outsourcing). These options are now likely to be challenged, as they do not necessarily deliver what authorities are looking for – best value for the users. Authorities recognize that they have to work in partnership with a range of organizations, including other local authorities and public agencies, to deliver fully joined-up services in their areas. Having opted for the partnership route, a choice has to be made whether to partner with public sector bodies, whether to partner with private, voluntary or social enterprise sectors, or whether to opt for a combination of them all. Central guidance emphasizes that partnering and collaboration is not an optional extra; in many situations, it is the only way modern services can be provided.

Social capital and asset-based community development

The principles of developing community action and personal skills contained in the WHO's Ottawa Charter highlight the importance of building 'social capital'. The Health Development Agency's book *Social Capital for Health: Issues of Definition, Measurement and Links to Health* (Morgan and Swann, 2004) demonstrates that the scientific literature is scattered with varying definitions of social capital, but most refer back to the work of Pierre Bourdieu (1986), James Coleman (1988) and Robert Putnam (1993), each bringing his own particular disciplinary perspectives to the concept. Bourdieu defines social capital in terms of social networks and connections. He posits that an individual's contacts within networks result in an accumulation of exchanges, obligations and shared identities that, in turn, provide potential support and access to resources. Coleman emphasizes the idea that social capital is a resource of social relations between families and communities. Putnam defines social capital as a key characteristic of communities. In his definition, social capital extends beyond being merely a resource to include people's sense of belonging to their community, community cooperation, reciprocity and trust, and positive attitudes to community institutions that include participation in community activities or civic engagement. Morgan and Swann observed that, while each of these authors describes social capital through a different disciplinary lens, their common thread relates to the importance of positive social networks of different types, shapes and sizes in bringing about social, economic and health development between different groups, hierarchies and societies. This is important in the context of partnership and collaboration between individuals, communities, organizations and government departments in working together to improve health and wellbeing.

In the report 'A Glass Half-Full: How an Asset Approach can improve Community Health and Well-Being' (Foot and Hopkins, 2010), the authors tell us that asset approaches are not new. Local politicians and community activists will recognize many of the features of asset-based working. However, their use as a method by which to challenge health inequalities is a relatively recent development in the UK.

Foot and Hopkins explain that the asset approach values the capacity, skills, knowledge, connections and potential in a community, rather than only seeing the problems that need fixing and the gaps that need filling. The more familiar 'deficit' approach focuses on the problems, needs and deficiencies in a community – such as deprivation, illness and health-damaging behaviours. It designs services to fill the gaps and fix the problems. As a result, a community can feel disempowered and dependent; people can become passive recipients of services, rather than active agents in their own and their families' lives.

Foot and Hopkins tell us that the asset approach is a set of values and principles and a way of thinking about the world. It:

- identifies and makes visible the health-enhancing assets in a community;
- sees citizens and communities as the co-producers of health and well-being, rather than the recipients of services;
- promotes community networks, relationships and friendships that can provide caring, mutual help and empowerment;
- values what works well in an area;
- identifies what has the potential to improve health and well-being;

- supports individuals' health and well-being through self-esteem, coping strategies, resilience skills, relationships, friendships, knowledge and personal resources; and
- empowers communities to control their futures and create tangible resources such as services, funds and buildings.

Foot and Hopkins believe that, while these principles will lead to new kinds of community-based working, they could also be used to refocus many existing council and National Health Service programmes. They tell us that the need for a people-centred and partnership way of working takes on added importance with the assets approach. This is a locality-based or outcome-based way of working, where silos and agency boundaries are not helpful; it is a people-centred and citizen-led approach. Joint investment in community building and sustaining social networks will bring benefits to all partner agencies. But it requires:

- an emphasis on prevention and early intervention;
- outcomes improvement through co-production with families and communities;
- a different model of leadership in partnerships;
- a lead by voluntary and community organizations, social enterprises and community networks by shifting their perspective towards community asset building; and
- a pivotal role for councillors, making visible the assets in their communities and supporting communities to develop their resources and thrive.

However, Foot and Hopkins point out that this research also shows that building wellbeing and improving social capital are rarely articulated as explicit outcomes of neighbourhood working or service design.

Co-production

The issue of partnership between people, communities and public sector organizations has also become important in government thinking about new ways of delivering and governing services, and is often described as co-production. Boyle *et al.* (2006) state that 'co-production' has emerged as a general description of the process whereby clients work alongside professionals as partners in the delivery of services. Boyle and Harris (2009) define co-production as meaning delivering public services in an equal and reciprocal relationship between professionals, people using services, their families and their neighbours. They say that, where activities are co-produced in this way, both services and neighbourhoods become far more effective agents of change. The central idea in co-production is that people who use services are hidden resources, not drains on the system; and that no service that ignores this resource can be efficient.

The people who are currently defined as users, clients or patients provide the vital ingredients that allow public service professionals to be effective. They are the basic building blocks of our missing neighbourhood-level support systems – families and communities – which underpin economic activity, as well as social development. Co-production shifts the balance of power, responsibility and resources from professionals to individuals, by involving them in the delivery of their own services. It is recognized that 'people are not merely repositories of need or recipients of services', but are the very resource that can turn public services around. Co-production also means unleashing a wave of innovation about how services are designed and delivered, and how public goods are acquired, by expecting professionals to work alongside their clients. It is central to the process of growing the core economy. It fosters the principle of equal partnership, and offers to transform the dynamic between the public and public service workers, putting an end to 'them' and 'us'. Instead, people pool different types of knowledge and skills, based on lived experience and professional learning.

In 2010, the Big Society was introduced as a flagship policy forming part of the legislative programme of the Conservative–Liberal Democrat Coalition Agreement. The Big Society is about helping people to come together to improve their own lives. It is about putting more power in people's hands – a massive transfer of power from Whitehall to local communities. There are three key parts to the Big Society agenda:

- *Community empowerment*: giving local councils and neighbourhoods more power to take decisions and shape their area;
- *Opening up public services*: public service reforms will enable charities, social enterprises, private companies and employee-owned cooperatives to compete to offer people high quality services; and
- *Social action*: encouraging and enabling people to play a more active part in society.

Anna Coote (2010) says that, when people are given the chance and treated as if they are capable, they tend to find they know what is best for them, and can work out how to fix any problems they have and realize their dreams. Bringing local knowledge, based on everyday experience, to bear on planning and decision-making usually leads to better results. Evidence shows that, when people feel they have control over what happens to them and can take action on their own behalf, their physical and mental wellbeing improves. While Coote says understanding that people have assets, not just problems, is a good start, she points out that not everyone has the same capacity to help themselves and others, and that how much capacity we have depends on a range of factors. A combination of social and economic forces, working across and between generations, results in some having much more and others much less. While these inequalities persist, people who have least will benefit least from the transfer of power and responsibility, and are at risk of being systematically excluded from any benefits that arise.

Coote believes that equality matters a great deal and the implications for the Big Society are profound, because she sees it weak on the structural links between economy and society.

Partnership working for health and wellbeing

Boydell *et al.* (2007) found that there are many models of partnership working, serving many and sometimes overlapping purposes (see, for example, Asthana *et al.*, 2002, Health Development Agency, 2003; Lasker and Weiss, 2003). Boydell *et al.* have developed a model (Figure 9.1) that seeks to demonstrate how, with effective processes and a favourable context, partnership working can lead to a reduction in inequalities. The model is intended as a way to conceptualize the benefits that may accrue through the developmental stages of the partnership, including those 'soft' or intangible ones that are not taken into account in other frameworks. In particular, it tries to capture the benefits that can 'spin off' at each stage and which may not be perceived as related to the partnership.

There is now ample evidence that health is determined by a broad range of determinants, including socioeconomic and environmental factors (Dahlgren and Whitehead, 1991; Evans *et al.*, 1994; Marmot and Wilkinson, 1999; Graham, 2000). Boydell *et al.*'s model acknowledges the strength of the existing evidence of these causal relationships and the fact that changes in these factors can impact on levels of inequalities in health.

On the far left of Figure 9.1, the model shows how various statutory agencies work alongside community, voluntary and private sector organizations to address the particular aspects of social and economic policy for which they are accountable or in which they have a particular interest. For many issues, working independently of one another is appropriate. However, where organizations face intractable problems that they cannot address on their own they often form partnerships (Audit Commission, 1998). In discussing their model, Boydell *et al.* say that – under favourable conditions, and once a partnership forms and begins to meet – partners connect with one another and develop relationships. Furthermore, they begin to connect one another to other networks outside the partnership. This is indicated in the first circle in the model moving from left to right. Based on the relationships formed, partners

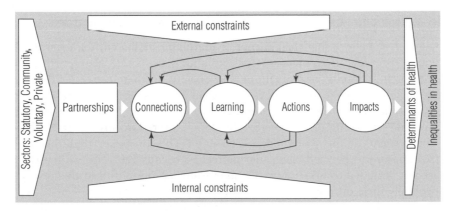

Figure 9.1   A model of the benefits of partnership

Source: Boydell *et al.* (2007), reproduced with the permission of the Institute of Public Health in Ireland.

start to get to know each other, to learn about each others' organizations and to gain an understanding of each others' agendas and work. They may develop a more holistic understanding of local communities' needs. They begin to develop trust. This is reflected in the second circle. As a result of this knowledge, understanding and trust, they may begin to act differently. They find that it helps them to do their jobs better, to meet their own organizations' agendas and to help others to meet theirs. They may find ways of tweaking resources or influencing others to achieve a broader goal. Finally, in the fourth circle, these developments can lead to more effective projects, programmes, improved service delivery and strengthening of communities.

However, Boydell et al. point out that there may be negative or unintended consequences. A range of barriers to progress in partnerships has been identified in the literature, many of which were raised by participants in this research (Balloch and Taylor, 2001; Glendinning et al., 2002; Sullivan and Skelcher, 2002; Bauld et al., 2005). The model includes these as internal and external constraints. Internal constraints are those factors that are inherent to the partnership itself, such as conflict between partners and the time-consuming nature of collaborative work. External constraints are those things that are beyond the control of the partnership but which impact on its ability to achieve its goals. These may include changing and conflicting policies, availability of resources and the political climate.

The model presents the benefits of partnerships arising in a linear fashion. However, Boydell et al. explain that the arrows between the circles indicate that this is highly iterative. Benefits may spin off at any stage in the model and may not be perceived by outside observers as being attributable to the partnership. Most partnership evaluation frameworks fail to identify these. One of the objectives behind developing the model was that it would provide a framework for how to measure partnership performance. Boydell et al. have developed indicators to assess performance along each stage of the model; that is, the connections, learning, action and impacts of partnerships.

Inter-sectoral partnerships, the knowledge economy and intangible assets

Boydell et al. believe that the concept of intangible assets within a knowledge economy provides a framework for explaining the value that partnerships create for individuals, organizations and society. In their paper (2007), they have introduced what they believe is a novel approach to assessing the value of partnerships as a form of governance, and consider their value from the perspective of 'intangible assets' (Sveiby, 1997, quoted in Boydell et al., 2007) in the context of the 'knowledge economy'. This proposes that the health sector appears to be inefficient and ineffective because current evaluations of it are not designed to take intangible assets into account, and in this respect it is probably little different from most other public services.

For organizations that emphasize the importance of knowledge as an intangible asset, the main strategy becomes one of enabling rather than controlling (Sveiby, 2001, quoted in Boydell et al., 2007). Such a strategy is aimed at improving what Sveiby refers to as people's 'capacity-to-act', either inside or outside the organization. All organizations are located in and interact with external communities, where they act as organizational nodes in larger social systems.

Boydell *et al.* think it is time to pay more attention to the ability to produce future value, rather than focus on past performance.

Outcomes-based partnership working

In Durham University's School of Medicine and Health paper (2008), 35 studies were selected that focused, at least to some extent, on partnership working and public health outcomes. Many of the studies look at the impact of health action zones. The review found that, while there is a plethora of literature testifying to the importance of partnership working, less emphasis has been placed upon the value of partnerships themselves in regard to their purpose in achieving better outcomes in improved health and support for recipients of interventions and/or services. The review concluded that, as the majority of the literature on partnership working focuses on the process and structure of partnerships, there is very little information on whether they are achieving their desired outcomes.

In March 2010, the Scottish Government published Briefing Paper 6 (McGuire, 2010). This was the first in a series of publications arising from the IS/Scottish Centre for Regeneration (SCR) collaborative project, which focuses on 'Embedding an Outcomes Approach in Community Regeneration and Tackling Poverty'. McGuire found that there is a growing consensus that the public sector ought to place greater focus on priority outcomes, delivered in more innovative and cost effective ways. Central to this will be the need to reassess approaches to partnership working. As part of this, the public sector undoubtedly needs to become more 'hard nosed' about partnership working and what it delivers.

McGuire believes that an 'outcomes approach' has the potential to provide significant leverage for delivering 'step change' in the quantity, quality and sustainability of outcomes achieved within communities. The focus will be on achieving enhanced outcomes in more effective ways through partnerships that are properly designed, empowered and accountable. The 'collaborative gain' analysis is seen to provide a number of useful insights into how the public sector can potentially deliver 'more with less' in order to achieve the priority outcomes that matter for communities. The key characteristics of an 'outcomes approach' are summarized as: results-focused; evidence-based; client-centred; joined-up; and early intervention/prevention.

Working in and managing partnership

Williams and Sullivan (2007) state that the motivations inducing individuals and organizations to work together are complex and diverse. Some are external and stem in part from government's attempts to coordinate and integrate the design and delivery of public services – sometimes referred to as 'joined-up' government – and evidenced in a variety of interventions, including statutory duties, policy instruments, financial and other incentives.

They say that the advantages of partnership lie in increased efficiency, better use of limited resources, tackling complex problems, enhancing learning and innovation, and improving the potential for inclusive and participative governance. Other motivations and drivers are internal to individuals and organizations. Practitioners and managers promote forms of cooperative behaviour for personal, professional or work-related reasons. For instance, many professionals are driven by altruism and believe that the public interest or client needs should be at the centre of public service organization, demanding integrated and coordinated frameworks of service planning and delivery. Some organizations consider exchanging and sharing resources to achieve jointly agreed purposes and benefits, to be more efficient in the use of resources, reduce transaction costs, and share risks and uncertainty about the future.

McGuire (2010) explains that 'collaborative gain' describes a situation where partnership working brings about added value benefits that could not have been achieved by the individual partner organizations operating on their own. In short, it is about achieving 'more than the sum of the parts'. He believes that collaborative gain rarely occurs by chance. Rather, the 'gain' anticipated must be clear and specific, and planned for in advance. Crucially, he believes that the anticipated gain to be achieved through working in collaboration with other organizations should outweigh the inevitable costs and challenges that can arise from partnership working. In terms of the outcomes approach, this will typically mean designing partnership working around the desired and agreed outcome. Subsequent planning ought to flow from this central focus.

Williams and Sullivan (2007) tell us that there are clearly costs and benefits to different forms of collaborative working. These need to be identified, understood and subjected to close scrutiny. The benefits of collaboration are potentially attractive and include sharing ideas, knowledge and resources to achieve, collectively, synergies that individual organizations would not be able to produce acting independently. Collaboration offers organizations the opportunity of influencing others to behave differently and cooperatively, and the process can be beneficial in terms of building trusting relationships and social capital.

In seeking to achieve collaborative gain, McGuire says that there is a wide variety of design options available concerning the type of partnership structure. This can range from the largely informal to the highly formalized. Regardless of the type of partnership structure selected, however, a key point of consideration will always relate to ensuring that appropriate accountability mechanisms are built into the partnership governance arrangements.

Williams and Sullivan believe that managing in collaborative environments is materially different from that in other forms of organizing and demands different approaches, behaviours and cultures. Practitioners, managers and other actors who assemble together to pursue joint strategies and action must learn and practise leadership and management skills that are different from those they have acquired and become familiar with in single organizations. The challenges they face are often daunting because of high levels of complexity, problems of multiple accountabilities and dispersed power relationships. In the face of often lengthy and tortuous decision-making processes, it is easy to revert to individual and organizational self-interest. But the benefits of collaborative working – particularly in its more developed forms in terms of synergy and co-production – are highly rewarding. Significantly, McGuire summarizes the shift in partnership culture, partly brought about by the outcomes approach, to be a move from:

- self-sufficiency to interdependency;
- fragmentation to integration;
- a service focus to an outcome focus;
- discrete accountability to mutual accountability;
- an agency focus to a customer focus.

Drivers for partnership working

Clarke and Stewart (1997) and the Audit Commission (1998) argue that collaboration is driven:

- by the need to deal with the proliferation of wicked issues (i.e. difficult problems often involving complex interdependencies);
- by the need to design new relationships with people and communities, and to formulate effective ways of engaging with them;
- by the desire to give expression to community leadership;
- by the need to deliver coordinated services because of the fragmentation of public bodies and agencies;
- as a bid for new or enhanced resources;
- to stimulate more creative approaches to problems;
- to align services provided by all partners with the needs of users;
- to influence the behaviour of the partners or of third parties in ways that none of the partners acting alone could achieve; and
- to meet a statutory requirement.

Other motivations can be traced to external factors. For instance, in the UK central government is particularly proactive in promoting a collaborative approach through a mixture of statutory regulation and general exhortation. Gray (1989), however, does not view government insistence on partnership working as a strong driver. He suggests that working together may improve the quality of solutions, as there is a greater capacity and capability brought to bear on the problem. Creative solutions to issues may be the result, and creative thinking may have greater influence on meeting the needs client groups. This is a benefit together with the potential to develop better relationships and use resources more effectively by reducing duplication.

The characteristics that support or hinder effective partnership

Cameron and Lart (2003) identify the factors that support or hinder joint working between health and social care. These can be summarized as:

- organizational factors (organizational differences, personalities involved, strong management and professional support);
- cultural and professional factors (trust and respect, different professional philosophies and ideologies); and
- contextual factors (political climate, constant reorganization, financial uncertainty).

Snooks *et al.* (2006), in a similar review of the evidence concerning the effectiveness of services delivered jointly by health and social care providers, identified a number of barriers to successful joint working, including:

- lack of investment in service planning, training, team development and leadership – particularly at the start of such a venture;
- unclear leadership channels;
- variable management structures, and different terms and conditions for staff; difficulties with roles and boundaries – particularly unequal power relationships, and inadequate communication channels.

On the positive side, good practice was identified as:

- investing in leadership;
- commitment of partners;
- integrated and flexible management structures;
- agreement about purpose;
- supportive environment, including suitable institutional structures;
- satisfactory accountability arrangements and appropriate audit and assessment;
- effective communication;
- shared decision-making; and
- a relaxation of boundaries – structural, organizational and financial.

There are circumstances when partnership working is not appropriate, and one example is when there is unclear demarcation in terms of who should tackle the issue and be responsible for the overall leadership. The so-called 'wicked issues' may fall into this category because of their complexity. Gray (1989) suggests that collaboration may not be appropriate if there are fundamental ideological differences, significant disparities in power, a history of antagonism and a failure of the partners to work together in the past. The cost of the partnership must also be consistent with the outcomes, and too great a cost will be a barrier. Boundaries – either in terms of geography, or organizations – may prove insurmountable. Partnership in the wellbeing of older people or children and young people, for example, should have the overall goal and shared concern of improving the quality of life and wellbeing for these groups.

Partnership and leadership

Williams and Sullivan (2007) found from their research that the leadership function in collaborative arenas needs to reflect shared responsibilities; complex systems; diversity; contested, diverse and fragmented sources of power; and divergent value systems and cultures. Leadership behaviour needs to inspire, nurture, support and communicate with individuals, teams and networks across and within different organizations. It is likely that traditional approaches to leadership, which focus on the specific actions of leaders, will not be appropriate in collaborative situations. Also, importantly, there is a need to focus on processes and skills that do not always reside in formally dedicated leaders. Hence the need to consider more dispersed and catalytic forms and approaches.

Partnership in practice

As the authors of this chapter, we have researched the wide range of literature on collaboration and partnership working. Having worked in the area of health and wellbeing for many years, we have experienced the practical challenges of setting up partnerships and making them successful. In our academic work, we have also studied partnerships and provided facilitation in bringing people together to think through how they can enter into the new and challenging working environment. People and organizations contemplating partnership often come from a wide range of sectors, backgrounds, professions and cultures. They are charged with different roles and responsibilities; are subjected to different social, economic and financial pressures; and are accountable in different ways to governing bodies and the recipients of their services.

We have found that, where partnerships are struggling or are not being as effective as they should be, the following areas often need attention:

- a strengthening of the overall relationships;
- clearer ownership and commitment to partnership working from the parent organizations;
- stronger governance arrangements and terms of reference, with clear accountability, and delegated authority of the board and its members;
- agenda driven by a jointly owned and focused action/delivery based business plan;
- a clear sense of purpose and a shared vision, with agreed aims, objectives and measures to help assess the progress and performance of the partnership and its members against its agreed deliverables, outputs and outcomes; and
- better inter-agency and community-wide engagement and communications.

The one thing our experience tells us is that we forget at our peril that setting up, managing or participating in partnerships is about managing and delivering change. Even given the supportive rhetoric often surrounding collaboration, one must look out for, and deal with, the barriers that will come in a number of forms and need to be unlocked or overcome. These barriers can take many forms:

- understanding – seeing and hearing what we want to, closed minds to new ways of working and others' views;
- emotional – risk averse, fear and uncertainty;
- cultural – tradition, lack of creativity and imagination;
- organizational – lack of commitment or support, centralized, insular; and
- cognitive – poor communications, inadequate information, rumour and myth.

Such barriers need to be anticipated, and identified. Engagement, open debate and creativity must be encouraged. The provision of time, training and support are essential. Recognizing and managing the transition from where you are to where you need to be, and dealing with difficult organizational cultures are important aspects of change management in the context of setting up new partnerships.

Effective communications in any organization are essential and should be geared to contribute to four things:

- creating a shared and jointly owned view of the future through engaging and communicating on strategy, mission and vision;
- integrating effort and commitment, and helping people to understand and position themselves in terms of their role, contribution and responsibilities in the partnership;
- nurturing and maintaining the health of the partnership – creating trust, removing prejudice and supporting collaboration, openly discussing problems, seeking solutions and celebrating success; and
- providing accurate and timely information up, down and between organizations for better understanding, leadership, decision-making and service delivery.

Conclusion

Partnership working toward health and wellbeing is firmly cemented as a central theme in both policy and practice. The public, private and third sectors have gained experience of joint working and collaboration in recent times but, from the research and reviews of practice, there is still much to learn and do to harness the clear opportunities partnership working offers to improve services and reduce inequalities. The range of factors affecting wellbeing means that many bodies – public sector, private sector and third sector – must be involved in any policy, programme or project to improve wellbeing. This inevitably means that inter-sectoral collaboration – to use the term coined by the Health for All 2000 movement – is of the essence. Or, put in other language, effective partnership working is the lynchpin of wellbeing.

Bibliography

Asthana, S., Richardson, S. and Halliday, J. (2002) 'Partnership Working in Public Policy Provision: A Framework for Evaluation', *Social and Policy Administration*, 36(7): 780–95.

Audit Commission (1998) 'A Fruitful Partnership: Effective Partnership Working'. London: Audit Commission.

Balloch, S. and Taylor, M. (2001) *Partnership Working: Policy and Practice*. Bristol: Policy Press.

Bauld, L., Judge, K., Barnes, M., Benzeval, M., MacKenzie, M. and Sullivan, H. (2005) 'Promoting Social Change: The Experience of Health Action Zones in England', *Journal of Social Policy*, 34(3): 427–45.

Bourdieu P. (1986) 'The Forms of Capital', in J. Richardson (ed.), *Handbook of Theory and Research for the Sociology of Education*. New York: MacMillan.

Boydell, L., Rugkasa, J., Hoggett, P. and Cummins, A. (2007) *Partnerships: The Benefits*. Dublin: Institute of Public Health in Ireland.

Boyle, D., Clarke, S. and Burns, S. (2006) 'Hidden Work: Co-Production by People Outside Paid Employment', Joseph Rowntree Foundation paper, June. York, UK: Joseph Rowntree Foundation.

Boyle, D. and Harris, M. (2009) *The Challenge of Co-Production: How Equal Partnerships between Professionals and the Public are Crucial to Improving Public Services* (NESTA and NEF).

Cameron, A. and Lart, R. (2003) 'Factors Promoting and Obstacles Hindering Joint Working: A Systematic Review of the Research Evidence', *Journal of Integrated Care*, 11(2): 9–17.

Clarke, M. and Stewart, J. (1997) *Handling the Wicked Issues: A Challenge for Government*. Birmingham: University of Birmingham.

Coleman J. (1988) 'Social Capital in the Creation of Human Capital', *American Journal of Sociology*, 94(Suppl.): S95–S120.

Coote, A. (2010) *Ten Big Questions about the Big Society and Ten Ways to Make the Best of It*. London: New Economics Foundation.

Dahlgren, Göran and Whitehead, M. (1991) *Policies and Strategies to Promote Social Equity in Health*. Stockholm: Institute for Futures Studies.

Deputy Prime Minister's Strategic Partnering Taskforce (2006) *Guide: Rethinking Service Delivery, Volume 3, Public/Public Partnerships*, June.

Dowling, B., Powell, M. and Glendinning, C. (2004) 'Conceptualising Successful Partnerships', *Health and Social Care in the Community*, 12(4): 309–17.

Durham University (July 2008) 'Partnerships in Public Health: A Healthy Outcome? Summary Findings of a Systematic Literature Review', Durham University, School of Medicine and Health.

Evans, R., Barer, M. and Marmor, R. (1994) *Why Are Some People Healthy and Others Not? The Determinants of Health of Populations*. New York: Aldine de Gruyter.

Foot, J. and Hopkins, T. (2010) 'A Glass Half-Full: How an Asset Approach Can Improve Community Health and Well-Being', March. London: Improvement and Development Agency, Healthy Communities Team.

Glendinning, C., Powell, M. and Rummery, K. (eds) (2002) *Partnerships, New Labour and the Governance of Welfare*. Bristol: Policy Press.

Graham, H. (ed.) (2000) *Understanding Health Inequalities*. Buckingham: Open University Press.

Gray, B. (1989) *Collaborating*. San Francisco: Jossey-Bass.

Health Development Agency (2003) *Working Partnership Book 1*. London: Health Development Agency.

Lalonde, M. (1974) *A New Perspective on the Health of Canadians*. Ottawa: Information Canada.

Lasker, R.D. and Weiss, E.S. (2003) Broadening Participation in Community Problem Solving: A Multidisciplinary Model to Support Collaborative Practice and Research, *Journal of Urban Health*, 80(1): 14–47.

Marmot, M.G. and Wilkinson, R.G. (eds) (1999) *Social Determinants of Health*. Oxford: Oxford University Press.

McGuire, A. (2010) 'Achieving Outcomes through Collaborative Gain', Scottish Government Briefing Paper 6, March, focuses on 'Embedding an Outcomes Approach in Community Regeneration and Tackling Poverty'. Improvement Service (IS)/Scottish Centre for Regeneration (SCR).

McMurray, R. (2007) 'Our Reforms, Our Partnerships, Same Problems: The Chronic Case of the English NHS', *Public Money and Management*, 27(1): 77–82.

Morgan, A. and Swann, C. (2004) *Social Capital for Health: Issues of Definition, Measurement and Links to Health*. London: Health Development Agency.

Putnam, R.D. (1993) 'The Prosperous Community: Social Capital and Public Life', *American Prospect*, 13: 1–8.

Snooks, H., Peconi, J. and Porter, A. (2006) *An Overview of the Evidence concerning the Effectiveness of Services delivered jointly by Health and Social Care Providers and Related Workforce Issues*. Cardiff: WORD.

Sullivan, H. and Skelcher, C. (2002) *Working across Boundaries. Collaboration in Public Services*. Basingstoke: Palgrave Macmillan.

Sveiby, K.E. (1997) *The New Organisational Wealth: Managing and Measuring Knowledge-Based Assets*. San Francisco: Berrett-Koehler.

Sveiby, K.E. (2001) 'A Knowledge-Based Theory of the Firm to Guide Strategy Formulation', *Journal of Intellectual Capital*, 2(4): 344–58.

WHO (1986) 'Ottawa Charter for Health Promotion', First International Conference on Health Promotion, Ottawa, 21 November 1986, WHO/HPR/HEP/95.1.

Williams, P.M. and Sullivan, H. (2007a) 'Learning to Collaborate: Lessons in Effective Partnership Working in Health and Social Care', October. Cardiff: NLIAH.

Williams, P.M. and Sullivan, H. (2007b) 'Working in Collaboration: Learning from Theory and Practice'. Cardiff: NLIAH.

Drugs Policy: A Case Study for Applying the Wellbeing Framework

Richard Pates

This chapter describes how the use of mind altering substances is universal and has brought benefits to many, but has also caused serious problems – in part, the result of attempts to control use through legislation. Current prohibitionist legislation is shown to run counter to the Ottawa Charter (WHO, 1986) and the Human Rights Act. A case is made for the reform of drug policy which acknowledges that the War on Drugs is not working and that drug use for many people enhances their wellbeing.

Introduction

The term 'drugs' is used widely not only for psychoactive substances, but also for those such as pain killers, antibiotics and chemotherapy agents, which are part of the medical armamentarium. Brian Inglis (1975), the social historian and journalist, stated: 'We take drugs for two reasons; either to restore ourselves to the condition we regard as normal – to cure infections or to take away pain; or to release us from normality – to enable us to feel more lively, or more relaxed; to alter our mood, or our perceptions': this has turned out to be true. Interestingly, drugs that have been developed or have evolved as major components of our pharmacopeia – such as opiates, cocaine, amphetamines, ketamine, and barbiturates – have not only provided benefit to humankind, but have also, on occasion, been the agents of misery and death. It is clear, therefore, that we need to look at the context and the way in which drugs are used. It is not necessarily the inherent nature of the drug itself that makes it 'dangerous' or problematic.

When considering wellbeing, it is important to remember that psychoactive substances (drugs, alcohol, tobacco, and so on) are an important part of many people's lives and, for some, a factor in their perception of wellbeing. The use of drugs varies from occasional recreational use to dependent use. Recreational use may be part of leisure activities akin to taking wine with a meal, which is harmless. Very heavy, dependent use of drugs or alcohol may lead to the destruction of the individual, and can also be extremely damaging to communities that become centres of dealing or heavy use. However, we do not tend to discriminate between different drugs and different types of use. In western societies, alcohol is usually seen as part of the fabric of society, and the majority of the population use alcohol recreationally with little disapproval. In those same societies, any form of illicit drug use is frowned upon, even though it may be safer and cause less harm to individuals and society than alcohol. So, where alcohol may be perceived as contributing to wellbeing, drugs rarely are – despite the fact that for some people they clearly do.

It seems likely that all drugs that are used recreationally, with the possible exception of tobacco, were originally exploited for purposes other than their mind altering capability, although drugs also play a part in community wellbeing – whether alcohol at a wedding reception or as used in religious ceremonies.

It appears that wherever the climate is suitable for the production of plants, there is a potential for the cultivation of species with psychoactive properties, or for the cultivation of plants that can be used in the production of such substances. Cannabis, for example, grows naturally in many parts of the world, as well as being extensively cultivated in some areas. The opium poppy has a wide distribution, including in temperate climates where is has been cultivated as a garden plant for many years. This is the same plant that is used in the production of opium and its derivatives: codeine, morphine and heroin. It is the most powerful analgesic known to humankind, but is also seen as the scourge of many cultures: street heroin has had, and continues to have, a major impact on communities. In many parts of the world, plants are grown specifically for the production of alcohol – such as the extensive cultivation of grapes for wine, barley for beer and sugar for rum. Alcohol is probably the most widely used psychoactive substance and, for many, its use is non-problematic; but it also causes major health problems through excessive use (p. 167). Attempts have been made to control alcohol use; for example, the gin laws in Britain in the 1750s, and prohibition in the United States in the 1920s and 1930s. There is currently a strong movement in the UK to try to tackle the epidemic of alcohol-related harm through measures such as unit pricing and restricting availability.

Siegel (1989) has described the need for mind altering drugs as the fourth biological drive after food, sleep and sex. We know that, historically, drugs have been used for centuries. Indeed, the use of the opium poppy was known to the ancient Greeks; and it is suggested that cocaine was found in the burial sites of ancient Egypt.

Alcohol has been used for thousands of years. It is produced as a result of deliberate fermentation of fruits and grains, but it also occurs naturally from the interaction of sugars contained in fruit and the yeasts that are found on their skins. There have been reports of elephants becoming drunk having consumed fermented fruit – a truly fearsome prospect, putting drunken teenagers into perspective! In the Bible, Noah is said to have 'lain uncovered' after drinking too much wine, and we know the parable of the wedding at Caanan where Jesus turned water into wine. So, alcohol has been part of the social fabric of society for many thousands of years. It has an important role in both Christian and Jewish culture. It has no place, however, in Islamic tradition.

In Britain in the seventeenth, eighteenth and nineteenth centuries, opium was widely available and was one of the few effective remedies for pain relief and the control of diarrhoea. It was also used to calm 'fractious' children. In 1864, the Registrar General voiced concern that the incidence of death from opiate poisoning was higher in children than in any other age group. Opium was available over the counter in many stores and was a constituent of a number of patent remedies, some of which are still available today (e.g. Dr Collis Browne's Chlorodyne). The town of Ely was surrounded by water up until the nineteenth century and was known for its high consumption of opium. The opium was used as a remedy for rheumatism and for the 'ague' (i.e. malaria), which was then prevalent. Shop counters in Fenland towns were regularly loaded on Saturday nights with three or four thousand vials of laudanum (opium dissolved in alcohol). In Spalding in Lincolnshire, in the 1860s drug sales averaged approximately 127 grains per head of population and one druggist in Ely sold 3 hundredweight of opium in a single year (Berridge, 1999). Interestingly, as Berridge points out, once the fens were drained, the high consumption of opium ceased.

Heroin was first synthesized from morphine in 1898 and was marketed by the German drug company Bayer as a drug to relieve coughing. Opiates do have a powerful anti-tussive action, and it is said that the most powerful cough mixtures are those that contain codeine, a derivative of opium. As with many other medications in the nineteenth century, heroin was advertised as curing a wide range of ailments.

The invention of the hypodermic syringe in the 1850s led to widespread use of morphine by injection as a putative cure for many conditions. By the 1880s, there was a growing awareness of both the potential for the transmission of infection by shared injecting equipment and of dependence on the drug. The people affected did not resemble the current image of the dependent opiate user. In Paris, in the late nineteenth and early twentieth centuries, middle-class women known as *morphineuses* would meet to inject morphine to relieve boredom. Lady Diana Cooper, a famous British society beauty, would intermittently inject morphine when she was bored, leading her husband Duff Cooper to hope that she wouldn't become a *morphineuse* (Ziegler, 1981).

Cocaine is another drug that is widely used in many parts of the world now and, because of the high profits to be made from it, is associated with violence and crime. However, when it was first synthesized in 1860 it was seen as a useful local anaesthetic, and also as a stimulant drug. It became acceptable with corporations such as Coca-Cola, whose famous product originally contained it. Sigmund Freud was an enthusiast for cocaine and wrote a paper in 1884, 'Über Coca', in which he eulogized cocaine for its beneficial effects. He saw it as a panacea for many ills and considered that it did no harm. He even advocated it as a cure for morphine addiction, asserting that it did not substitute one addiction for another – 'it does not turn the morphine addict into a *coquero*; the use of coca is only temporary'. He later retracted his enthusiasm for cocaine when he realized its addictive potential.

The fictional detective Sherlock Holmes was also a *habitué* of the drug, using a hypodermic syringe. In recent times, cocaine (especially in the form of crack) has not only been associated both with high rolling, successful people such as rock stars and bankers, but also with prostitution as a means of paying for the costly drug.

Aldous Huxley, in his science fiction novel *Brave New World* (1932), wrote of people taking holidays from their present reality by using the drug 'soma'. Instead of physically going away, they could travel in imagination by taking soma, an interesting and plausible use of drugs with a long action!

The above is not intended to be a complete social history of drug use but, rather, some illustrative examples of drug use across cultures and history.

Why do we use drugs?

What is apparent is that drug use needs a number of conditions to flourish:

Availability: this does not imply legality. If a substance is not available, there is no use of it. In Europe we do not see the use of kava, a narcotic root used in the Pacific Islands; or betel nut chewing, a drug that is extremely widely used across Asia. This is mainly due to their lack of availability.

Acceptability: this does not have to be a society-wide acceptance but acceptance from one's peer group or the group with which one wishes to be identified. This explains the use of sex and glamorous images for the advertising of tobacco and alcohol.

A role for the drug: for example, a pleasant psychoactive effect, or as a solution to unpleasant conditions. Examples of this include the use of coca leaves by indigenous South American peoples to enable them to work at altitude and in extreme conditions, the use of opium by the fen dwellers, and the rise of alcohol misuse during the industrial revolution. These issues will be discussed later in the chapter.

As indicated, drugs have been used throughout history and appear to be used universally across cultures. There appears to be a human drive for altered states of consciousness, whether for the sake of stimulation or for relaxation, and these may be over and above the specific effects of drug use. We know, for example, that for some people there is a great need for sensation seeking, which may express itself in bungee jumping, riding fast motorcycles or seeking out dangerous situations. For these people, sometimes, stimulant drugs can have similar effects. Drugs such as opiates can have a very calming, relaxing effect on the mind and have the effect of distancing problems, whether physical, emotional or financial. Habitual opiate users have described the sensation as being 'wrapped in cotton wool'. Interestingly, it seems likely that different people may be drawn to different drugs because of the specific effect that a particular drug gives them.

In the mid-eighteenth century in Britain, there arose what became known as the gin craze, where the quantities of gin consumed – mainly by working class people – led to major problems with public drunkenness. Hogarth's engraving 'Gin Lane', exemplifies this with the chaos that supposedly came from heavy gin drinking, including a nursing mother dropping her baby on its head (Figure 10.1). The consumption of gin became a significant issue and a number of laws, the Gin Laws, were enacted to try to counter it. These were probably among the earliest attempts at harm reduction by use of the law, which did eventually reduce the consumption of gin nationally. What is interesting to note is that the rise of gin drinking corresponded with the rise of the industrial revolution and the increased movement of people from the land to live in the expanding cities, where they not only lived in squalid premises, but also had appalling working conditions. One can speculate that one of the reasons for the heavy drinking was as a way of coping with the intolerable conditions of everyday life. The wellbeing of the working class poor must have been at a low ebb; the cheap way of escape was through strong alcohol.

With alcohol misuse there is a complex relationship between young people starting to drink and the development of tolerance. It is clear that drinking in many cultures, especially in twenty-first-century Britain, has become something

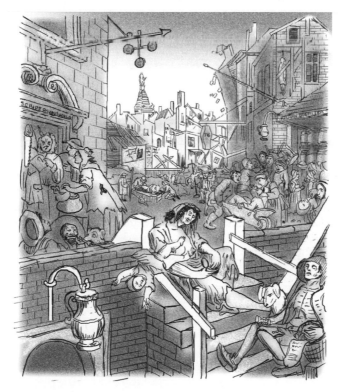

Figure 10.1   Gin Lane cartoon

Source: Steve Haslam (derived from William Hogarth's 1751 engraving), reproduced with permission of the British Museum.

that is not only embedded in society, but is also seen as a problem. But when young people start drinking, usually at an inappropriate age, they may not like what they are drinking because of the adult, sophisticated nature of the taste of beer and spirits. The first time that beer is drunk, it may be perceived as being too bitter to enjoy but this abreaction will be overridden by the psychological necessity of being part of the beer drinking culture. It is for this reason that, in an attempt to encourage young people to drink alcohol, the drinks industry has developed 'alcopops' which, while tasting sweet and harmless, and thus acceptable to young people (Mosher and Johnsson, 2005), in reality may contain up to 5 per cent alcohol by volume. The effects of needing to overcome the initial negative experiences of a drug are even more pronounced with tobacco, where, until one becomes tolerant, smoking it is a very unpleasant experience with no gains other than social acceptability. The initial effects of nausea and dizziness would have a strong aversive impact were it not for the social acceptability and the social cachet gained from the habit.

There is also the role of expectation which, for the user of a drug for pleasurable purposes, is its sought after specific effect. So, for the injector of heroin there will be an expectation of 'a rush' (an intense feeling of brief duration following within seconds of administering the drug), followed by the opiate induced reverie known as being 'stoned'. However, if these effects are not expected, as in the case of a post-operative patient using a self-administered morphine pump, the equivalent 'rush' may be experienced as extremely unpleasant and the opiate induced 'stoned' state disliked because it renders normal functioning difficult. So, there is a large expectation effect with drugs, depending on what is sought from their use.

Society's view of drugs does change. A good example is the use of morphine in the late nineteenth and early twentieth centuries by middle-class women who could obtain the drug over the counter at pharmacies. These drug users were not seen as problematic, unlike modern day young street drug users ('smack heads') who are dependent on a very impure form of the drug. Yet, in both cases it is the same substance – morphine, or a derivative of morphine such as heroin – that is being used. Another example is tobacco, which is becoming increasingly unacceptable socially in the developed industrialized nations, whilst its use in countries such as China and Africa is burgeoning. The unacceptability of smoking in the developed nations has recently been signalled by banning it in public places such as offices, public houses and restaurants. These changes have been introduced gradually over a protracted period of time and have been widely welcomed and accepted. However, prohibition of tobacco use appears not to work and is not on any country's agenda, with the possible exception of Finland.

Prohibition as a means of control

There have been many attempts throughout history to control the use of drugs. Some have already been mentioned and others will be discussed. What is interesting is that they rarely have the desired effects, and may have unwanted collateral effects. One of the early attempts to control the use of gin in eighteenth-century Britain arose from the concern about the effect on working-class people. Daniel Defoe, writing in 1728 about the craze for drinking cheap spirits which afflicted London's poor, opined: 'common people get so drunk on a Sunday that they cannot work for a day or two following. Ney [sic], since the use of 'Geneva' (gin) has become so common many get so drunk they cannot work at all, but run from one irregularity to another 'til at last they become arrant rogues' (Defoe 1728, quoted in Linnane, 2008).

The reasons for the problem were partly the cheapness of gin and its availability. Britain was producing a glut of grain and distilling it into gin was vastly profitable, as taxes on the home produced product were low. The duty was only 2d per gallon and sellers did not need a retail licence, the drink being sold in thousands of premises of various degrees of respectability. In 1725, there were 6187 outlets in the capital, excluding the City of London and Southwark: 220 years later a London that had increased greatly in size had only 4,000 pubs (Linnane, 2008). Among the poor, almost everyone drank gin; men, women and children – and even infants. It was used as an anaesthetic to silence starving children and a food substitute for starving parents. A cheap skinful bought a few hours escape from misery (Linnane, 2008). In an attempt to control these problems, various pieces of legislation were enacted. In 1729, a licence fee of £20 was imposed for retailing spirits and the duty was raised from 2d to 5 shillings per gallon. These measures were found to be unenforceable and were repealed in 1733 – and followed by another outbreak of drunkenness and disorder.

In 1736, the Gin Act was introduced, which required a £50 licence fee for retailing spirits. This led to rioting, and a number of people paid to inform on those who subverted the Act were stoned to death by a mob. The result was that, in seven years, only three licences were purchased. However, it led to a vast increase in informers and, in a period of two years, there were 12,000 cases brought for contravention with 5,000 convictions (Linnane, 2008). In 1751, another Gin Act reduced the number of gin shops and increased taxes once more, so that within a few years the annual British consumption had fallen from 11 million gallons per year to 1 million. It is interesting to note that the gin craze was almost entirely restricted to London. It had a very serious effect on working-class Londoners, but was eventually contained through legislation and taxation, and also through the widespread use of paid informers.

During this period, parliament was dominated by gentleman farmers, in many cases the same people who were making substantial sums of money from their grain distilled into gin. Thus, there was a political dimension to the gin craze. Another cause of the growth of the distilling industry in Britain was the high tariff imposed by the government on imported spirits.

Another example of the attempt to use legislation to control alcohol use was the Volstead Act in 1920 that led to prohibition in the US. The Act did not achieve its objective of significantly reducing alcohol consumption and it was repealed in 1933. In the 13 years of its existence, however, an illicit liquor industry developed that was controlled by organized crime with much associated violence.

Musto (1997) suggests that prohibition failed not because it did not reduce alcohol consumption but, rather, because it did not gain the overwhelming support of the American people, a necessary prerequisite for the successful prohibition of a drug. He goes on to say that it is customary to judge the impact of prohibition by the amount of alcohol that was consumed, or by comparing the lives saved from reduced deaths from cirrhosis compared with those shot by gangsters and prohibition agents. The most serious impact of prohibition, however, was the half century of resistance to dealing with alcohol problems that followed the repeal of the Volstead Act. In 1934, per capita alcohol consumption was slightly less than one gallon of alcohol per year (the lowest recorded level in American history). It then rose until it reached a peak in 1980 of 2.8 gallons per capita.

A parallel can be drawn between the involvement of organized crime during the era of alcohol prohibition and the current control of the illicit drugs market in contemporary society. Most countries have laws prohibiting the use and sale of certain drugs – usually the opiates; and some, such as Singapore, retain the death penalty for dealing in these drugs. However, this appears not to be a disincentive for people to carry on dealing in and using these drugs. In modern Iran – a country which has produced large quantities of opium – despite harsh government and religious prohibition, the extent of opiate use is alarming. There is a major epidemic of addiction, including the injection of heroin and the many consequences associated with the latter.

For several decades, America has been publicly waging 'a war on drugs' that appears not to have had any impact on drug producers. The current situation in Mexico – a major source of drugs for the American market – includes a level of violence from the drug cartels and the law enforcement agencies that appears to be unstoppable and out of control. An article in the *New York Times* on 23 October 2010 (Malkin, 2010) reports that, since the Mexican government began its crackdown on drug cartels four years ago, Ciudad Juárez has become one of the most violent cities on earth. Murder fuelled by the drug trade has become so commonplace that residents are no longer easily shocked. The article reported the deaths of 13 people shot in a raid on a house – a raid that appeared to be caused by feuding rival gangs.

The level of opiate and other drug use has fluctuated throughout history, as has that of alcohol. Current legislation aimed at attempting to control opiate and cocaine use has resulted, unsurprisingly, in large sums of money being made by organized crime. There are also links with terrorist and insurgency groups which, in many cases, have generated income from dealing in drugs. A similar scenario is posited in Afghanistan for the Taliban, who ironically were originally supported by the American government. The CIA also had a role in drug dealing in South East Asia during the early years of the Vietnam War (McCoy, 2003). The inconsistency of approach adopted by the US government is well-illustrated by the case where it was proposed to get farmers in South America to grow coffee beans rather than coca, yet agreement on a minimum price for coffee beans necessary to persuade the farmers to do this was vetoed, thus dooming the project to failure.

In the UK, the main legislation for the control of drugs is now the Misuse of Drugs Act 1971. This piece of legislation is nearly forty years old and is out-of-date, as the drug problem in the UK in the 1960s was in no way comparable to the situation that now prevails. British drug policy in its modern form dates back to the Hague Convention of 1912. The aim of the Convention was to bring about the gradual suppression of the abuse of opium, morphine and cocaine by limiting manufacture to 'medical and legitimate purposes'.

The Defence of the Realm Act 1914 was an attempt to ensure that the effectiveness of the armed forces and staff working in munitions manufacturing was not compromised by excessive consumption of intoxicating substances. It was the Defence of the Realm Act that first introduced restricted licensing hours for the sale of alcohol and made the gift or sale of intoxicants – defined as any sedative, narcotic or stimulant – to a member of the armed forces with the intent to make them drunk or incapable: an offence punishable by a sentence of prison for up to six months.

In 1926, a committee was established under Sir Humphrey Rolleston that introduced what became known as 'The British System', which meant that the treatment of drug addiction was deemed to be a matter for the medical profession, and that the prescribing of drugs of dependence to addicts by doctors was considered an appropriate measure. This was contrary to the prevailing thought in the United States, where drug use was criminalized and the forced treatment of addicts was carried out. In 1931, a register kept at the Home Office listed only 245 addicts throughout the UK. In 1934, a central collective record was established (or, as it became known, an Addicts Index). Because most of the addicts obtained their supplies from doctors and heroin was not available on the street, it was relatively easy to calculate the total number of addicts. The number of addicts nationwide was 700, in 1935. The Addicts Index was kept by the Home Office until 1997 and its demise has been regretted by many people working in the field, as it is now no longer possible to count the number of people dependent on drugs (Spear, 2002).

Throughout the 1950s and 1960s there were relatively few notified addicts. In 1968, notification to the Home Office became statutory and the number on the Addicts Index in that year was 1729. This shows that the problems of serious drug use in Britain then were insignificant compared with the position at the time of writing, when there are thousands of people addicted to opiates and cocaine. During the period up to the late 1960s, much of the treatment of addicts and the prescribing of heroin was carried out by general practitioners; often in a fairly uncontrolled way, with certain notorious doctors over-prescribing and thereby creating a black market in heroin. In a letter to the *British Medical Journal* in 1967, Dr John Hawes reported that some of his patients told him that powdered heroin had appeared for the first time on the black market as an alternative to the usual tablets obtained on doctors' prescriptions. This was the first indication of an increasing problem of heroin use in the UK, and led to the second Brain Report, which changed the format of treatment but also foreshadowed the Misuse of Drugs Act (1971) (Spear, 2002).

As part of the Misuse of Drugs Act, the Advisory Council on the Misuse of Drugs (ACMD) was established. This advised the government on drug policy and on the system of classification of drugs. The Act comprised three classes:

- Class A, the most dangerous, including heroin and cocaine;
- Class B, which included cannabis, amphetamines and barbiturates; and
- Class C, which included non-prescribed benzodiazepines, which were then beginning to become a problem.

From the start, there were anomalies in these classifications, which were intended to be based on the level of danger to life. For example, LSD (which was popular in the 1960s as a powerful hallucinogenic drug) was included as a Class A drug, even though it was not life-threatening, albeit having potentially serious psychiatric consequences. Magic mushrooms (which grow in many parts of the UK in fields, parks and gardens) were also classified as Class A drugs. This meant that if they were passed to another person, even with no money changing hands, this was classified as dealing in Class A drugs – potentially punishable with a life sentence!

Legislation that could improve the conditions and wellbeing of people who use drugs

There are various pieces of legislation and international agreements that could help to improve the conditions and wellbeing of people who use drugs. The Ottawa Charter (WHO, 1986) aimed to improve health through community action. It identified five approaches to health promotion:

- building healthy public policy;
- creating supportive environments;
- reorienting health services;
- strengthening community action; and
- developing personal skills

Current drug policy, with its focus on prohibition, contains elements that run counter to these principles. It can hardly be construed as health promoting. Supportive environments are not created for those with the problems associated with drug and alcohol use, and health services are generally not oriented to treating such people. Community action is often more about restriction rather than health, and personal skills have often been overlooked in terms of working with substance users. Pates (1995) gives examples of how all these could be changed to comply with the Ottawa Charter. So, for example, building healthy public policy could be reflected in changes in drug regulation, and also in removing barriers to treatment and locations where help is provided. There have been some changes recently, with a few police forces becoming more sympathetic and diverting users into treatment. But there is still a long way to go before anything like compliance with the Ottawa Charter precepts is achieved.

The recognition and sympathetic treatment of the mental health problems that so often accompany drug use – the well-recognized dual diagnosis problem – could provide an example of creating a supportive environment, as proposed under the Charter.

In 2000, the Human Rights Act became law in the UK. It was an incorporation of the 1950 convention for the Protection of Human Rights and Fundamental Freedoms (better known as the European Convention on Human Rights). Article 5 of the Convention states that:

Everyone has the right to liberty and security of person. No one shall be deprived of his liberty save in the following cases and in accordance with a procedure prescribed by law.

Included in these exemptions is the 'lawful detention of persons for the spreading of infectious diseases, of persons of unsound mind, alcoholics, drug addicts or vagrants'. Thus, after making progress in making human rights an important issue and a legal issue, it then marginalizes some of the most vulnerable people in our society – seeming not to accept that the mentally ill, people with drug and alcohol dependence, and the homeless are part of our community (Pates, 2000).

The Secretary General of the United Nations, Ban Ki-Moon, stated in 2008: 'There will be no equitable progress in HIV prevention so long as some parts of the population are marginalised and denied basic health and human rights – people living with HIV, sex workers, men who have sex with men and injecting drug users.' In many countries, drug use – especially injecting drug use – is so circumscribed by the criminal justice system that human rights are often infringed. This may, for example, include denying or limiting access for drug users to substitution therapy, incarcerating large numbers of users, and measures that specifically work against good public health policy. This may go across a whole range of behaviours from denying treatment to people; cruel, inhuman and degrading treatment; and even executions and destruction of crops where no adequate market for substitute crops is first arranged.

Reforming drug policy

There has been a growing awareness over the last few years among some very influential people that current drug legislation requires radical change. Some, including the former Chief Constable of the North Wales Police, have called for the legalization of all drugs.

A declaration on drug policy was agreed at a recent conference in Prague, ('Urban Drug Policies in the Globalised World', Prague, 2010), where representatives of municipal governments from around the world met with experts in the fields of drug regulation, policy, treatment, prevention, harm reduction and research. The declaration proposed seven principles for the assessment of drug policies:

1   *No size fits all*: This principle stated that, despite the need to operate within national drug policies and the international drug control regime (as defined in three United Nations drug conventions), this does not require uniformity of drug policies at local level. It is important that

local policies take advantage of all the freedoms available within national legal frameworks for experimentation and innovation.

2   *Realism is the key*: A drug free world is an unrealistic aim, and harmful if set as an ultimate goal. However, it is beneficial and realistic to aim to diminish the harms related to drug trafficking and use as much as possible, by reducing the non-medical consumption of drugs by means of prevention, treatment and regulation.

3   *Human rights apply to ill people, in particular*: The World Health Organization (WHO) defines drug addiction as a disease with multiple causes. There is no scientific justification and no ethical principle to support the criminalization of a disease or for citizens being deprived of their human rights because they are ill. The human rights and dignity of those afflicted by drug addiction should be recognized and protected by all those involved in drug policy and its implementation at all levels.

4   *Public health and public safety concerns must not be seen as contradictory*: Often, intervention in the drug field is interpreted as a compromise between public safety and public health, suggesting that these are in opposition. This runs counter to scientific evidence and experience in the field. Interventions that are effective in public health terms are also beneficial for the safety of communities, because the health of a community is a vital part of its perceived safety.

5   *Evidence-based decisions only*: The problems of illegal drugs and their harmful impacts are many and their interactions are very complex, influenced by a range of factors. These factors relate not just to psychiatry and criminology, but also to other factors: genetic, biological, social, religious/spiritual, political and economic, among others. Many of the simplistic ideas presented as self-evident may prove – and have, in some cases, already been proven – to be false, or even harmful. All decisions in the field of drug policy, as in other areas of policy, should be firmly rooted in scientific evidence.

6   *Evaluation and monitoring*: The monitoring and evaluation of interventions is widely recognized as a *sine qua non* for the successful implementation of any intervention, programme or policy. Only those drug policies that involve evaluation as an inherent component can be assessed and constantly improved.

7   *Constant and improving mutual information flows between local, national and international levels of drug policy through common voice*: The assessment, evaluation and development of national and international norms should increasingly be seen from the local perspective, and be influenced by that perspective. Such a process may be fostered by the creation of a global platform for networks of cities that are dealing with drug policies, which already exist in some countries and regions.

The Prague Declaration shows a shift in thinking towards recognition of the need for sensible evidence-based policies that reflect local need. Another important document), 'After the War on Drugs: Blueprint for Regulation', published by the Transform Drug Policy Foundation (2009), identifies several scenarios for regulating the supply and use of drugs within a legal framework. In its foreword it states, 'The vast majority of the horrific harms associated with drug use – crime, HIV and other blood borne infections, violence, incarceration, death – are clearly fuelled by the prohibitionist drug policies our governments pursue.'

This report highlights the inadequacy of current drug laws and puts forward a number of scenarios that look at different models of regulation of drug markets. It works from the tenet that current prohibition policies on drugs have increased the harm that is done both to users and to society. The report offers a number of *regulatory* options for each class of drug, a scenario far removed from the free-for-all situation that prohibitionists fear and use to argue against the possibility of a legalized model. Some countries have already decriminalized drug possession. This is the case in Portugal, where this has not lead to an increase in hard drug use or to its becoming a destination for drug tourists. The accent is now on treatment, rather than penal sanctions. A number of countries in South America (including Argentina, Brazil, Ecuador, Bolivia and Mexico) have moved, or are moving, towards the decriminalization of drug possession and a public health model to prevent and treat the misuse of drugs. They are no longer able to tolerate the damage done by the War on Drugs (Transform Drug Policy Foundation, 2009). Given the number of recorded deaths in Mexico in 2009/10 associated with the drug trade and the efforts of the police and army to contain it, this seems a sensible and timely approach.

Wellbeing

If happiness is, as suggested by Albert Camus, the simple harmony between a man and the life he leads, one can imagine that for some people the use of a substance to make them feel better is part of that happiness – be it a glass of chilled Chablis as a relaxant after work, a tablet of ecstasy in a club, or even a syringe of heroin. They all give pleasure, but can lead to problems if taken in excess. Even the American Declaration of Independence includes the inalienable right for the pursuit of happiness – rather ironic given America's current stance on people pursuing pleasure through mind altering substances!

When thinking of wellbeing and its association with the use of mind altering substances, it is helpful to consider the three components of the mind:

- affect: dealing with emotion and mood,
- cognition: dealing with the thought processes and intelligence, and
- conation: the processes of driving, volition or how decisions made are put into action.

Psychoactive substances impact on mood and emotion (affect), stimulants produce feelings of wellbeing, confidence and happiness, and sedative drugs produce different feelings of relaxation, lethargy and reverie. Unless psychoactive substances are taken unknowingly (such as in drug rape cases), taking such a substance involves a series of intellectual actions and decisions based on experience, knowledge and expectations; that is, cognition. The putting of those decisions into action requires a motivation, a volitional state that will override fears of the possible effects of the substance and of the consequences of use being illegal in order to achieve the desired state. So, it can be argued that the pursuit of happiness requires affective, cognitive and conative processes; this is particularly true if the pursuit of that happiness is associated with a specific decision to use a psychoactive substance to help achieve it.

Legislation on drug control has had many negative effects and has rarely been successful in restricting or controlling drug use. The Volstead Act in the United States, which brought in prohibition, resulted in deaths from poisoning from illicitly brewed liquor, large profits for organized crime and much violence associated with turf wars between rival criminal gangs. It did, however, lead to a decrease in the incidence of cirrhosis of the liver.

The prohibition of illicit drugs has been similarly ineffective in controlling their use. The War on Drugs, a concept introduced by President Nixon in the early 1970s, has not resulted in the elimination of drugs. Also, in the early days of the HIV epidemic, prohibition did nothing to limit the spread of the disease among injecting drug users. As an example of not creating supportive environments (Gillman, 1990), in the late 1980s New York had an estimated 200,000 heroin users, with an estimated number of over 50 per cent being HIV positive. A needle and syringe exchange programme was introduced but operated for only a short time before being discontinued. Conditions were imposed on the programme: only one sterile needle per visit per person was allowed, and no needle exchange could be sited within 1000 yards of a school – which severely hampered the programme's effectiveness from the start.

In a number of countries, the death penalty is still the punishment for 'drug trafficking'. In Singapore, there is a mandatory death penalty for anyone caught in possession of more than 15 grammes of heroin, 30 grammes of cocaine, or 500 grammes of cannabis – quantities that in other countries might count only for personal possession. In Thailand, in 2003, a 'war on drugs' was declared by the government that resulted in the judicial deaths of 2,800 people. One impact of this was a significant decline in people seeking treatment for drug problems (Barrett et al., 2009). In the UK – where cannabis has been, and still is, classified as a class B drug – the effect has been that the many thousands of non-problematic users (as well as those who use it as a palliative for conditions such as multiple sclerosis and certain cancers) run the risk of acquiring a criminal record if apprehended in possession of the drug. The likely impact of such a record on their lives and future careers is considerable.

The issues mentioned here are just a few examples of where the law, far from being helpful in controlling drug use and leading to improved wellbeing, may have devastating effects on people's lives and little impact on reducing drug use.

In the 1950s and 1960s, an American psychologist, Lawrence Kohlberg, developed a theory of moral development (Crain, 1985). Through giving children and adults ethical dilemmas to solve, he worked out a six-stage model of such development comprising three stages of morality: preconventional morality, conventional morality and postconventional morality.

Preconventional morality comprised:

- Stage 1: *Punishment and obedience* orientation – this involves the child obeying the rules simply because they are the rules;
- Stage 2: *Individualism and exchange* – where the child recognizes that there is not just one possible view but an identification of the right one as that which most serves their own self interest.

Conventional morality comprised:

- Stage 3: *Good interpersonal relationships* – children believe that people should live up to expectations of family and community, and behave in 'good ways';
- Stage 4: *Maintaining the social order* – there is a perception of the needs of wider society whereby laws must be obeyed, and authority respected; most people achieve this stage of moral development and get no further.

Postconventional morality comprised:

- Stage 5: *Social contract and individual rights* – this recognizes that questions might be asked about what sort of society is desired, and consideration may be given to the rights and values society ought to uphold;
- Stage 6: *Universal principles* – this recognizes that the law might not always be right and that the 'principles of justice require one to treat the claims of all parties in an impartial manner, respecting the basic dignity of all people as individuals'. This principle requires that a law should not be introduced that aids some people but hurts others.

Using this model, it can be seen that achieving societal wellbeing is a higher stage of moral development that should not involve the benefit of one member of society being to the detriment of another.

Conclusion

What this chapter has shown is that the use of psychoactive substances is not a peculiar aberration of a small proportion of society but, rather, a worldwide phenomenon that has been occurring for centuries. The reality is that most people derive pleasure and possibly benefit from this but, for a few, the harm caused is substantial and can be devastating. However, it is also clear that the effects of prohibition itself have an impact on quality of life and societal wellbeing, and can even have fatal consequences.

Health effects and mortality are not the only issues that affect those using drugs. Drug use can cause devastation in communities; and in relationships, particularly where children are concerned (ACMD, 2003), and lead to financial ruin. Alcohol can have similar effects. Despite the similarities between the potential damage of illicit drugs and alcohol, they are treated very differently under the law; this situation applies in most countries. In many countries, legislation is being passed or proposed to try to reduce the harm caused by alcohol – which, in many cases, includes trying to involve the alcohol industry. The situation with illicit drugs is very different, with many countries using draconian laws to attempt to limit use. These laws have clearly not only failed, but are also often contributing to diminished population wellbeing.

Drug use has escalated in most countries. As indicated, in the UK the number of problematic drug users has risen from a few hundred in the 1960s to many thousands in 2010. In the United States, drug use has escalated in similar ways, despite even stronger prohibitionist legislation and enforcement. Even in countries where drug dealing or possession may be punished by the death penalty, drug use has increased.

In the light of prohibitionist legislation that has not worked and a war on drugs that has compounded the problem, a radical reform of current policy is required – with serious consideration being given to legalization or, at least, decriminalization. If drugs were removed from the crime agenda and some system of regulated distribution of drugs was introduced, population wellbeing would improve in many ways. The one country in Europe that has decriminalized drug use is Portugal. When this was proposed, it was suggested that Portugal would become a destination for drug tourism and that it would become overwhelmed by a massive drug problem. This has not been the case: people have been directed into treatment, rather than prison, when a drug problem is recognized. Vastag (2009) reported that, in the five years following the change in the law, deaths from street drug overdoses dropped from 400 annually to 290, the incidence of HIV infection dropped from 1400 in the year 2000 to 400 in 2006; and that, instead of going to prison, addicts were going into treatment and were learning to control their drug use or come off drugs entirely. Although these indications are not themselves measures of wellbeing, it would not be unreasonable to imagine that the wellbeing of this group of people has improved immeasurably.

Bibliography

Advisory Council on the Misuse of Drugs (2002) 'The Classification of Cannabis under the Misuse of Drugs Act 1971'. London: Home Office.

Advisory Council on the Misuse of Drugs (2003) 'Hidden Harm – Responding to the Needs of Children of Problem Drug Users'. London: Home Office.

Advisory Council on the Misuse of Drugs (2005) 'Further Consideration of the Classification of Cannabis under the Misuse of Drugs Act 1971'. London: Home Office.

Ban, Ki-Moon (2008) 'Remarks on the Handover of the Report of the Commission on AIDS in Asia at United Nations Headquarters, New York, 26 March, Quoted in V. Barrett, C. Cook, R. Lines, G. Stimson, and J. Bridge (2009) *Harm Reduction and Human Rights: The Global Response to Drug Related HIV Epidemics*. London: International Harm Reduction Association.

Barrett, V., Cook, C., Lines, R., Stimson, G. and Bridge, J. (2009) *Harm Reduction and Human Rights: The Global Response to Drug Related HIV Epidemics*. London: International Harm Reduction Association.

Berridge, V. (1999) *Opium and the People: Opiate Use and Drug Control in Nineteenth and Early Twentieth Century Britain*. London: Free Association Books.

Beverley, R. (1705) *The History and State of Virginia in Four Parts*. London: R. Parker, Quoted in R. Rudgley (1998) *The Encyclopaedia of Psychoactive Substances*. London: Little Brown.

Carrell, S. (2010) 'Anthrax Contaminated Heroin Kills Drug User', *Guardian*, 10 February.

Crain, W.C. (1985) 'Kohlberg's Stages of Moral Development', in W.C. Crain, *Theories of Development*. New Jersey: Prentice-Hall: 118–36.

Freud, S. (1884) 'Über Coca, Centralblatt Für Die Ges', *Therapie*, 2: 289–314.

Gillman, C. (1990) 'After One Year, New York City's Needle Exchange Pilot Programme', *International Journal on Drug Policy*, 1(5): 19–21.

Huxley, A. (1932) *Brave New World*. London: Chatto & Windus.

Inglis, B. (1975) *The Forbidden Game*. London: Hodder & Stoughton.

Linnane, F. (2008) *Drinking for England*. London: JR Books.

Malkin, E. (2010) '13 are Killed as Gunmen Storm House in Mexico', *New York Times*, 23 October.

McCoy, A.W. (2003) *The Politics of Heroin: CIA Complicity in the Global Drug Trade. Afghanistan, Southeast Asia, Central America, Columbia*. Chicago: Chicago Review Press.

Mosher, J. and Johnsson, D. (2005) 'Flavoured Alcoholic Beverages: An International Marketing Campaign that Targets Youth', *Journal of Public Health Policy*, 26(3), September: 325–42.

Musto, D.F. (1997) 'Alcohol Control in Historical Perspective', in M. Plant, E. Single and T. Stockwell (eds), *Alcohol: Minimising the Harm*. London: Free Association Books.

Pates, R. (1995) 'The Effects of Policy Making on Harm Reduction: Whose Problem?', *International Journal of Drug Policy*, 6(1): 39–45.

Pates, R. (2000) 'Human Rights for Whom?', Editorial in *Journal of Substance Use*, 5(5): 207.

Prague Declaration (2010) Prague Declaration ('On the Principles of Effective Local Drug Policies'), *Addictology*, September supplement: 62–3.

Siegel, K.R. (1989) *Intoxication: Life in Pursuit of Artificial Paradise*. London: Penguin.

Spear, B. (2002) *Heroin Addiction Care and Control: The British System 1916–1984*. London: Drugscope.

Transform Drug Policy Foundation (2009) *After the War on Drugs: Blueprint for Regulation*. Bristol: Transform Drug Policy Foundation.

Vastag, B. (2009) '5 Years After: Portugal's Drug Decriminalization Policy Shows Positive Results', *Scientific American*. Available at http://www.scientificamerican.com/article.cfm?id=portugal-drug-decriminalization (accessed 11 April 2011).

WHO (1986) Ottawa Charter for Health Promotion, *Health Promotion International*, 1(4): iii–v.

Ziegler, P. (1981) *Diana Cooper: The Biography of Lady Diana Cooper*. London: Hamish Hamilton.

A Greatest Wellbeing Principle: Its Time Has Come

11

Paul Walker and Marcus Longley

This chapter draws out some of the main messages from the preceding chapters; identifies the key steps that the authors consider should be taken to advance the wellbeing agenda; gives a vision of how the NHS and other public services might be different in 25 years' time, if the wellbeing concept is widely adopted; identifies a seeming gap in the current deconstruction of wellbeing requiring focused research; gives a brief critique of the concept; and ends by emphasizing that wellbeing is much more than mere happiness and must be recognized as such.

Perspectives on wellbeing: a synthesis

As demonstrated in Chapter 1, over the last forty years there has been a growing salience of the wider/social determinants conception of public health. This – together with an increasing interest in the subjective elements of health, as manifest by the development of the health and medical outcomes movement – betokens a convergence of public health and wellbeing thinking, and agendas with the prospect of the latter replacing the former. One tangible benefit that would result, it is suggested, is the greater engagement of relevant agencies and disciplines in the form of partnership working, which is the key to delivering the wellbeing and inequalities agendas.

However, the perceived convergence of public health and wellbeing is merely part of a greater, more fundamental perception which is, as Chapter 2 suggests, that wellbeing is the unifying principle of all social policy and, as such, should be the yardstick by which all public policies, programmes and projects are planned and evaluated.

Far from being merely an interesting abstraction, wellbeing is readily measurable in both subjective and objective terms. A wide range of metrics are available, so it is now possible to monitor the impact of particular schemes. Crucially, by using both objective and subjective measures in this process, it should be possible to ensure that social justice is not compromised and that the problem of adaptation (p. 33) is avoided.

For a variety of reasons, outlined in Chapter 3, the wellbeing framework has not been embraced by the NHS. To achieve its adoption – and there are very good reasons why it should be adopted – it will have to satisfy the needs of each of the three structural interests within the NHS: management, health care professionals and patients/general public. This will not be easy. It means, among other things, that the concept must be seen as both robust and measurable, and that managers and professionals must be prepared to think outside the traditional NHS box and overcome their own traditional perceptions and prejudices. Not an easy prescription.

Local authorities control many of the local drivers of wellbeing but have been slow to take advantage of this. To do so, and to fulfil their statutory duty to promote the economic, social and environmental wellbeing of their populations, they need to become better at integrating their own diverse services – particularly with the spatial planning function; and better at coordinating these services with those of other organizations, such as the Health Service (Chapter 4). Promoting community wellbeing should be seen as the prime objective of planning sustainable communities, as well as providing a platform for the active involvement of the general public in local governance as elements of the Big Society movement.

Recent surveys of children and young people in the EU and other developed countries give no grounds for complacency about the current state of wellbeing of this age group, or about how children and young people in the UK compare with those in neighbouring countries (Chapter 5). There is a growing realization that the state must intervene to safeguard the wellbeing of children, but evidence that this is declining suggests a failure of this state responsibility. The current policy approach to the wellbeing of young people is less clear-cut, with a widespread belief that they are, in large measure, the architects of their own ill-being and merit sanctions by the state to protect society from their deviant behaviour.

As the proportion of the population aged 65 years and over (Chapter 6) continues to grow, the wellbeing of this age group will increasingly affect the overall wellbeing of the population. There is evidence that their wellbeing is higher than that of any other age group, but this overall positive picture undoubtedly hides a pattern of variation in wellbeing between the younger members and the older ones, as well as between those who have to survive on a state pension and those with generous occupational and/or private pensions. Social isolation, cold homes, and failing physical and mental health are significant issues, particularly for those aged 85 years and over. These have a major impact on wellbeing and are likely to have an increasingly negative impact on overall population wellbeing as the proportion of this age group increases.

The promotion of wellbeing in the workplace (Chapter 7) is now well-established in the UK, with strong backing from the government. There is evidence from population surveys that an individual's experience in the work-place has a significant effect on their overall sense of wellbeing. So, the evolving wellbeing at work movement is important not only for the obvious reason of increasing productivity, but also as a means of improving employees' own wellbeing and as a platform for broadcasting the wellbeing concept beyond the workplace to the wider community.

Though community development has been widely promoted as a vehicle for community involvement and empowerment, Chapter 8 contends that it has been used by the public sector as a smokescreen for top-down executive action, with only a tokenistic nod towards community participation. The well-being framework, with a focus on both subjective and objective wellbeing, could be a mechanism for securing real community involvement and for facilitating co-production.

Though collaboration has been on the agenda in the UK since at least 1974, it has generated much more rhetoric than action. However, as Chapter 9 demonstrates, things are changing. Partnership working towards health and wellbeing is increasingly firmly cemented as a central theme in policy and practice for the public, private and third sectors. Yet, research and reviews of practice show there is still much to learn and to do in order to harness the clear opportunities partnership working between the wide range of agencies involved offers for the development of health and wellbeing agendas. Inter-sectoral collaboration – to use the term coined by the Health for All 2000 movement – plus the new framework of co–production are necessary components of such partnership working.

It is a fact, as Chapter 10 describes, that mind altering substances such as drugs and alcohol contribute positively to wellbeing for many people, and have done so since time immemorial. For many, their use is a necessity of living. Accepting this, and looking dispassionately and objectively at the evidence of the impact of current prohibitionist policy, would in our view reveal that any policy would be preferable in net wellbeing terms to the current one, and that some form of regulated legalization would have the greatest potential wellbeing gain to users and society in general.

Essential steps to progress

So, what are the minimum steps required to progress the wellbeing agenda?

What we are describing here is a fundamental shift in the way public policy is conceived and implemented. We are also looking for common ground between different political philosophies, in the belief that wellbeing has currency across the political spectrum. Change of this sort, on this scale, prob-ably requires us to look simultaneously at three ways of making progress:

- *Understanding*: We need to win the battle for hearts and minds: people in positions of power and influence need to understand what wellbeing means, and come to believe in it. This means addressing a variety of intel-lectual and motivational issues.

- *Incentivization and leadership*: The agents of public policy – all those staff in the public services who can make a difference – need to work with the grain of wellbeing, making decisions and delivering services in ways conducive to greater wellbeing. This requires a set of incentives, positive and negative, to incline people in the right direction. Such incentives need to recognize that people – especially in the public services – are usually motivated by a desire to do the right thing, rather than some crass desire to maximize their own personal benefit. So, we are looking here more at the nudge than the shove!
- *Empowerment*: Citizens – individually, in families, in the work place and in civic society – are probably the most powerful element in all this. People generally do not need help in understanding the value of wellbeing, but they may need support in realizing it, in removing unhelpful barriers, and in providing a level playing field.

In the light of this, we offer Ten Steps to Wellbeing. The staircase has many more than ten steps in total, but these are some of the first:

Understanding

- We need to be clear what we are talking about, and a common language is a key element in this. Agreement on measures of subjective and objective wellbeing to be used by all is crucial, together with a supporting research programme for development and refinement of these. The principle of the perfect being the enemy of the good is eminently applicable here. The measures chosen have to be good enough for their purpose, not perfect.
- A major programme of understanding and information for all public sector managers and workers is urgently required. A key element in this is the professionals, for whom the emphasis should be on the close connections between their normal professional practice and ethics, and the concept of wellbeing. As with all such approaches, key individuals need to be identified; followed by a process of 'cascading'. It should also become a standard core component of all management education programmes in the public services.
- The adoption of wellbeing by a significant number of local authorities in the UK as a central focus for policymaking and the delivery of local services to their communities thus providing demonstration sites.
- The preparation of Wellbeing Charters, containing key planning principles to be adopted in the development of sustainable new communities and as the platform for community development and empowerment generally.

Incentivization and leadership

- Wellbeing champions need to be identified in local government, the voluntary sector, the private sector and, of course, central government. The latter is almost certainly the most important, and the establishment of a Minister for Wellbeing based in the Cabinet Office and serving the Prime Minister and individual Secretaries of State would serve as an important marker of the importance of wellbeing. Adding the term 'wellbeing' in the titles of all state departments would signal the fact that all departments have, as an underlying objective, the improvement of wellbeing of a particular section of the population. So, restyling the Department of Health as the Department of Health and Wellbeing would send out a powerful message about the importance of wellbeing, and the relationship of health to the achievement of wellbeing. In the devolved nations, the approach should be basically the same, but the task should be somewhat easier, given their smaller size and clearer focus. The job of the champions is to explain and enthuse. It is also to encourage colleagues to look at what more could be done to promote wellbeing, and also at where services need to do less – where regulation and approach frustrate or even undermine wellbeing.

- There should be a statutory duty on all public sector organizations to undertake a wellbeing impact assessment on all policies, programmes and major projects, with a presumption that the voluntary and private sectors will also conduct impact assessments wherever possible and appropriate.
- 'Quality of Life Indicators' should be used by local authorities for objective analysis and measurement of general wellbeing through the use of local household surveys. This will mirror the proposal at a national level by the Coalition government to have a combined wellbeing data set prepared by the Office of National Statistics. The data should be scrutinized by local authority Wellbeing Scrutiny Committees to oversee the roll-out and application of the wellbeing function in all local authority services.

Empowerment

- There should be an increased level of public involvement and engagement with public service providers to achieve more efficient and effective ways of delivering better wellbeing outcomes for everyone. Work should be invested particularly in the most deprived communities, so that these can be equipped with the capabilities and receive the cooperation they need to tackle the challenges they face. This needs to embrace a wide variety of groups in the population, and different settings. For example, children in schools are already taking part in story circles and many other approaches to provide them with the means with which to enhance their own wellbeing: we need even more of this. In workplaces, employers need to do much more to allow staff to shape working practices to enhance their wellbeing: the economic and humanitarian cases for this are equally compelling.
- There should be an increased role for the voluntary sector in delivering services and running community facilities in the interests of improving wellbeing. Politicians of all persuasions have come to understand how civic society – however defined – is crucial in building resilience, self-help and mutual support. A focus on wellbeing provides additional incentive to get smart with this agenda: we are barely beginning to understand how the state can nurture this precious capacity in every community. The promotion of community-based initiatives and actions within existing or new

communities to establish Healthy Living Centres in premises that may include general practitioner group practice surgeries, health and community centres, secondary schools and leisure centres.

A vision of the future

Accepting wellbeing as the prime or underlying objective of all social policy – and, thus, as the unifying framework for all social policy – represents a paradigm shift with major implications for government and all public and voluntary sector organizations. One can only speculate on the degree to which policy discourse, political debate, partnership working, the role and power of general public and the way organizations and services are run would be changed.

For example, what might the NHS look like in this scenario?

Clinical care would be transformed, with a new focus on patients' own feelings and wishes, rather than those of the health care professionals. Instead of patient reported outcomes for a few procedures, patient determined outcomes for all procedures and interventions would be the norm, putting the patient firmly in the driving seat. Services would be genuinely developed in partnership with the communities they serve.

Collaboration with other agencies in promoting public wellbeing would be standard procedure, with sharing of budgets against common wellbeing objectives and with the full engagement of management and professional staff. The Department of Health would be a Department of Health and Wellbeing. The NHS would become the National Health and Wellbeing Service.

The only reliable guardians of the public wellbeing are the public themselves: at primary and secondary care levels, the public voice – democratically elected – must be heard and have primacy over the professional voice. So, in hospital trusts the board will have a majority of elected lay members with a corporate formal responsibility to safeguard and promote the wellbeing of patients and the local community. At primary care level, similarly, general practitioner consortia will have a governing body with a majority of elected lay members with, again, a corporate formal responsibility to safeguard and promote the wellbeing of patients. Primary care teams will also have a formal responsibility to promote the wellbeing of their practice populations through community development for wellbeing.

In recognition of the importance of subjective health and wellbeing, there will be a major commitment to palliative care not just for cancer patients, but for all patients with chronic illness. And it should be accepted that dying in hospital is a circumstance to be avoided whenever possible, and to be accounted for when it is putatively unavoidable.

The training of doctors and of all health care personnel would be much more focused on subjective health and an understanding of the importance of the subjective mental state not only as an outcome measure of health care delivery, but also as a factor affecting physical health and the response to physical therapies. The training of nurses, in particular, will need to be refocused, with more emphasis on the caring and subjective aspects of health care.

As for local government, if it were to implement its wellbeing powers fully and acknowledge that it controls many of the local levers for delivering wellbeing, it would, among other things, become much more corporate and much less departmental. It would devolve powers and finance to local communities – for example, through the creation and empowering of community councils or their equivalent.

A gap in our understanding of wellbeing

As outlined in Chapters 2 and 10, a rather surprising omission in the discourse on wellbeing is any reference to conation. There is consensus that wellbeing is a subjective state of mind, with distinct affective and cognitive components. But if, for example, an important element of an individual's wellbeing comprises achieving career goals in the course of their lifetime, without conation these goals would be mere thoughts with no prospect of achievement.

The whole empowerment movement, which has wellbeing gain as its prime objective, must be based on developing the will and power of those concerned. So, there is a clear need in our view for a coherent research programme aimed at exploring the role of conation in wellbeing and at applying the resultant understanding to, among other things, improving methods of empowerment.

A critique of wellbeing

There are some who question the whole basis of an approach that focuses on wellbeing or happiness. Sen and also Nozick, among others, have made major criticisms mainly relating to the issues of 'other goods', expediency, rights, agency, adaptation and the nanny state.

One could reasonably ask, as has Layard, what is so special about happiness compared with other good things. The answer, he suggests, is that happiness is the only experience that is self-evidently good: Man is programmed to enjoy experiences that are good for survival, which is why he has survived. So, the desire to be happy is a central feature of our nature.

Another objection is that adopting Bentham's Greatest Happiness principle is impractical and encourages expediency. However, where moral or legal considerations are in conflict, some overarching principle is required to provide a resolution. This is exactly what a greatest happiness rule provides and what a greatest wellbeing rule could provide in greater measure.

The principle is also criticized for putting ends before means. This is a misconception for, in taking a decision based on maximizing happiness or wellbeing, the whole sequence of feelings experienced by those affected – those experienced during the action (the means) as well as those that follow it (the ends) – are taken into account.

Another objection is that it does not start from human rights or desirable 'capabilities'. But, in selecting what human rights to consider, it is inevitable that the choice would be made on the basis of some rights being preferred because they are more conducive to human happiness and wellbeing. This makes happiness or wellbeing the underlying human right or 'capability'.

A further objection is that humans adapt and that, for example, some people can be happy even when external circumstances are harsh. People can even adapt, in part, to poverty. According to Sen, this might be used to justify leaving them in poverty and to subvert action to reduce inequalities. Accepting this objection the solution, as indicated in Chapter 2, is to ensure that both subjective and objective measures of happiness or wellbeing are used in all circumstances where adaptation is a risk.

Finally, there are those who might accept a greatest happiness or wellbeing principle as a private ethical guide, but reject its use for public policy. However, the concept of wellbeing has the useful capacity to appeal across the political spectrum, albeit for somewhat different reasons. For those on the right, the key thing is that it speaks to self-defined outcomes. Both elements of that are important: self-defined, because that privileges autonomy and not the 'nanny state'; and outcomes rather than means – again, allowing for self-determination. For those on the left, wellbeing appeals because it can be cast in terms of citizens' 'right' to self-fulfilment, regardless of wealth.

Interestingly, both right and left embrace the notion that wellbeing is, in part, determined by society. For those on the left, the focus tends to be on material circumstances and equality, and the role of the state in levelling the playing field; for those on the right, the rhetoric now ascribes causal power to family, institutions and the Big Society.

The UK Coalition government has started now to measure 'happiness' for these very reasons. In his recent book, entitled *The Big Society*, Jesse Norman (Conservative MP for Hereford and South Herefordshire) sets out the case for 'compassionate Conservatism' (Norman, 2010), and the role of happiness and wellbeing in that. In essence, it recognizes that atomized individuals generally will not find happiness, and that institutions such as the family, work, school and church are key elements in general wellbeing. The role of the state is to recognize its own inherent limitations to making people happy and to confine itself to supporting those other institutions, which can do much more.

So, wellbeing's focus on self defined outcomes helpfully makes the concept palatable to both right and left.

Johns and Ormerod (2007) point out that democratic decision-making already takes into account many desirable outcomes other than economic growth. They contend that the dichotomy presented by many proponents of the greatest happiness principle is a false one – that is, that use of gross national product implies a narrow, materialistic and self-centred view of welfare, while use of happiness indicators would imply a more holistic or ethical conception. They also suggest that the overriding of individuals' own judgements of what is good for them and makes them happy by remote policymakers who aver that they can prove that these judgments are wrong is both undemocratic and unattractively paternalistic.

To the philosopher Isaiah Berlin, the greatest happiness principle demonstrates the 'Ionian' fallacy – the tendency to prioritize one value above all others. Nowhere is this fallacy better satirized than in chapter 17 of Aldous Huxley's dystopian novel *Brave New World*:

> 'But I don't want comfort' [said John the Savage] 'I want God, I want poetry, I want real danger, I want freedom, I want goodness, I want sin.'
>
> 'In fact', said Mustapha Mond [World Controller for Western Europe] 'you're claiming the right to be unhappy ... Not to mention ... the right to be tortured by unspeakable pains of every kind.'
>
> There was a long silence.
>
> 'I claim them all,' said the Savage at last.

In conclusion, Richard Layard's words say it all:

> We are at the beginning of a major revolution in public values ... This points the way for a revolution in political philosophy ... We need a political philosophy which is intrinsically defensible but also internally consistent. Consistency means that if people use the philosophy in their individual lives, the result will be the society which the philosophy advocates. The principle of the greatest happiness satisfies this requirement ... The nineteenth century saw increased social responsibility; while the past 40 years have seen increasing individualism. We do not need a return to Victorian values, some of which were pretty gloomy. Instead, we need a philosophy which fully values happiness and enjoyment, but at the same time enjoins us to strive for the happiness of others (2009: 105).

Afterword: is happiness the same as wellbeing?

As indicated in Chapter 2, there are several related concepts in circulation – wellbeing, quality of life and happiness to mention the main ones – which mean more or less the same thing but, importantly, not quite the same thing. Richard Layard and others have majored on happiness and, in much of the discussion in this book, happiness and wellbeing have been used interchangeably, as if they were synonyms. However, it is important to acknowledge that, on analysis, happiness turns out to be a poor imitation of wellbeing because it has a weak or non-existent cognitive component, whereas the cognitive element of wellbeing is at least as important – arguably, more important – as the affective one. Aristotle defined the distinction between wellbeing and happiness 2,500 years ago.

Recent publicity about the coalition government's interest in constructing a wellbeing index has revealed a widespread misconception that wellbeing is the same as happiness – which is seen as a rather trivial, even comedic, concept. But as David Willetts, the responsible Minister, has commented, 'This is not about measuring happiness as it has been caricatured. Indeed, the key to progress in this subject – just as in real life – is to get beyond a preoccupation with happiness. Wellbeing is different. It is much more to do with the pursuit of external goals and happiness comes as a by-product of that. The Canadian provinces with the highest life satisfaction are the ones where there is most volunteering. Harvard psychologist Brian Little has put the point very pithily: 'what makes life worth living is not the pursuit of happiness but the happiness of pursuit.'

Or, put more prosaically and to quote Libby Purves, 'Politicians want to measure our happiness, but they need to distinguish between fulfilment and fleeting feelings'; and alluding to the evergreen comic and singer, Ken Dodd, 'The happiness he sings about cannot be unconnected with the fact that he is still honing new jokes, touring six-hour shows at the age of 84 and bathing in giggling applause. Work, achievement, an answering echo from humanity: all you need.'

To Cicero the health of the people was the highest purpose. We believe that, today, the wellbeing of the people, not its happiness, is the highest purpose.

Bibliography

Berlin, I. (1998) 'Does Political Theory Still Exist', in Henry Hardy and Roger Hausheer (eds), *The Proper Study of Mankind*. London: Pimlico: 78.

Griffiths, S. and Reeves, R. (2009) *Well-Being: How to Lead the Good Life and What Government Should Do to Help*. London: Social Market Foundation.

Huxley, A. (1932) *Brave New World*. London: Chatto & Windus: 237.

Norman, J. (2010) *The Big Society*. Buckingham: University of Buckingham Press.

Layard, R. (2009) 'Afterword', in Simon Griffiths and Richard Reeves (eds), *Wellbeing. How to Lead the Good Life and What Government Should Do To Help*. London: Social Market Foundation.

Little, B. (1998) 'Personal Project Pursuit: Dimensions and Dynamics of Personal Meaning', in P.T.P. Wong and P.S. Fry (eds), *The Human Quest for Meaning: A Handbook of Research and Clinical Applications*. Mahwah, NJ: Erlbaum.

Purves, Libby (2011) 'I'm Not in the Mood for Smiley "Happyology"', *The Times*, 11 April: 19.

Willetts, D. (2010) 'Happiness Is Not ... an Attack on Free Markets', *The Times*, 26 November: 38.

Index